The long-term treatment of functional psychoses:
needed areas of research

The European Science Foundation is an international non-governmental organization with its seat in Strasbourg (France). Members are Academies and Research Councils which are responsible for supporting scientific research at a national level, and which are funded largely from government sources. The term 'science' is used in its broadest sense to include the humanities, social sciences, biomedical sciences and the natural sciences with mathematics. The ESF has currently 48 members from 18 European countries.

The tasks of the ESF are to:

assist its Member Organizations to coordinate their research programmes and define their priorities;

identify areas in need of stimulation, particularly those of an interdisciplinary nature;

further cooperation between researchers by facilitating their movement between laboratories, holding workshops, managing support schemes approved by the Member Organizations, and arranging for the joint use of special equipment;

harmonize and assemble data needed by the Member Organizations;

foster the efficient dissemination of information;

respond to initiatives which are aimed at advancing European science;

maintain constructive relations with the European Communities and other relevant organizations.

The ESF is funded through a general budget to which all Member Organizations contribute (according to a scale assessed by country), and a series of special budgets covering Additional Activities not included in the main programme, to which only participating Organizations contribute. The programmes of the ESF are determined by the Assembly of all Member Organizations. Their implementation is supervised by an elected Executive Council, assisted by the Office of the Foundation which consists of an international staff directed by the Secretary General and located in Strasbourg.

European Medical Research Councils
a Standing Committee of the
European Science Foundation

The long-term treatment of functional psychoses

needed areas of research

Proceedings of a Workshop held in Villa Lante, Bagnaia
9–11 May 1983

Edited by T. Helgason

In collaboration with
E. E. Anttinen
B. Cronholm†
R. Daly
H. Hippius
E. A. Sand

† Deceased in 1983.

The right of the University of Cambridge to print and sell all manner of books was granted by Henry VIII in 1534. The University has printed and published continuously since 1584.

CAMBRIDGE UNIVERSITY PRESS
Cambridge
London New York New Rochelle
Melbourne Sydney

CAMBRIDGE UNIVERSITY PRESS
Cambridge, New York, Melbourne, Madrid, Cape Town,
Singapore, São Paulo, Delhi, Tokyo, Mexico City

Cambridge University Press
The Edinburgh Building, Cambridge CB2 8RU, UK

Published in the United States of America by Cambridge University Press, New York

www.cambridge.org
Information on this title: www.cambridge.org/9780521106108

First published 1985
First paperback edition 2011

A catalogue record for this publication is available from the British Library

Library of Congress Catalogue Card Number: 84-23149

Library of Congress Cataloguing in Publication Data
The long-term treatment of functional psychoses:needed areas of
research:proceedings of a workshop held in Villa Lante,
Bagnaia, 9–11 May 1983.
1. Psychoses
I. Helgason, T. II. European Medical Research Councils
616.89′1 RC512

ISBN 978-0-521-26628-4 Hardback
ISBN 978-0-521-10610-8 Paperback

CONTENTS

List of Participants vii

Introduction *T. Helgason* 3

I **Organisational Aspects of Long-term Treatment**

Classification of functional psychoses requiring long-term treatment *E. Strömgren* 9

Structural changes in psychiatric hospitals *N. Retterstøl* 15

Alternatives to hospitals: a field of promises and of not-yet answered questions *C. Perris* 25

The closing of mental hospitals in Italy and its impact on long-term treatment of functional psychoses *E. Torre* 39

Future developments in Italy *R. Misiti* 47

Optimal duration of long-term treatment in functional psychoses *R. Sadoun* 51

II **Patients Aspects of Long-term Treatment**

Needed areas of research in psychological treatments for functional psychoses *R. Daly* 59

Family therapy as part of the treatment of schizophrenia *Y. O. Alanen* 77

Milieu therapy in the long-term treatment of functional psychoses: needed areas of research *P. Vaglum and S. Friis* 89

Long-term treatment of functional psychosis with neuroleptics *R. Öhman and R. Axelsson* 101

Lithium and prophylaxis in manic-depressive illness *P. Vestergaard* 107

New perspectives in psychopharmacology *O. J. Rafaelsen* 115

Research implications of recent trends in the treatment of schizophrenia *L. Ciompi* 123

Long-term treatment of functional psychoses in childhood and adolescence *J. Appelboom-Fondu* 139

Functional psychosis in old age *C. Müller* 145

Chronicity and hospitalization: can the vicious circles be broken? *E. E. Anttinen* 151
Social network and the long-term course of mental disorders – research needs *H. Katschnig and T. Konieczna* 163

III Public Health Aspects of Long-term Treatment
Introduction to public health aspects of chronic illness and long-term treatment *H. Häfner* 177
Evaluation of long-term community care for patients with schizophrenia *H. Häfner and W. an der Heiden* 183
Case registers for monitoring treatment outcome in chronic functional psychoses *D. Walsh* 197
Social disability and chronic mental disorder *R. Giel, A. de Jong, C. J. Slooff and D. Wiersma* 207
The neglect of the patient with chronic functional psychosis: the need for further research *R. G. Priest, P. Raptopoulos and M. L. Chan* 217
Suicides and functional psychoses *N. Juel-Nielsen* 235
Interaction with families *J. Leff* 241
Cost-effectiveness analysis *D. Goldberg* 247
Consumption of services – European aspects *J. H. Henderson* 255

Index 261

PARTICIPANTS

Professor Yrjö O. Alanen
Department of Psychiatry
Institute of Clinical Sciences
University of Turku
20 700 Turku 70
Finland

Professor Erik E. Anttinen
Department of Public Health
University of Tampere
Žäkäriuk. 3
33 520 Tampere 52
Finland

Dr J. Appelboom-Fondu
Département de psychiatrie
Hopital Académique Erasme
Université Libre de Bruxelles
Route de Lennick 808
1070 Bruxelles
Belgium

Professor F. Baro
Department of Psychiatry
Catholic University of Leuven
Leuven
Belgium

Professor Luc Ciompi
Director
Socio-Psychiatric University Clinic
Murtenstrasse 21
CH-3010 Bern
Switzerland

Professor L. B. Cronholm
Karolinska Hospital
Solnavägen 1
S-104 01 Stockholm
Sweden

Professor Robert J. Daly
Department of Psychiatry
University College Cork
Cork Regional Hospital
Wilton, Cork
Ireland

Professor R. Giel
Psychiatrische Kliniek
Academisch Ziekenhuis Groningen
Oostersingel 59
Postbus 30.001
9700 RB Groningen
The Netherlands

Professor David Goldberg
Department of Psychiatry
University of Manchester
The University Hospital of
South Manchester,
West Didsbury
Manchester M20 8LR
United Kingdom

Professor Heinz Häfner
Direktor
Zentralinstitut für Seelische Gesundheit
6800 Mannheim J5
Federal Republic of Germany

Professor W. an der Heiden
Zentralinstitut für Seelische Gesundheit
Postfach 5970
6800 Mannheim J5
Federal Republic of Germany

Dr John H. Henderson
Regional Officer for Mental Health
World Health Organization
Regional Office for Europe
8, Scherfigsvej
DK-2100 Cophenhagen Ø
Denmark

Professor H. Hippius
Ludwig Maximilians Universität München
Psychiatric Clinic
Nussbaumstrasse 7
8000 München
Federal Republic of Germany

Professor Nils Juel-Nielsen
Institute of Psychiatry
Odense University Hospital
5000 Odense C
Denmark

Dr Heinz Katschnig
Allgemeines Krankenhaus der Stadt Wien
Psychiatrische Universitätsklinik
Lazarettgasse 14
A-1097 Wien
Austria

Dr Julian Leff
Assistant Director
MRC Social Psychiatry Unit
Friern Hospital
Friern Barnet Road
London N11 38P
United Kingdom

Professor Raffaello Misiti
Istituto di Psicologia
Consiglio Nazionale delle Ricerche
509 Via dei Monti Tiburniti
00157 Roma
Italy

Professor H. J. Möller
Psychiatrische Klinik der Technische
Universität
Rechts der Isar
Ismannigerstrasse 22
D-8000 München 80
Federal Republic of Germany

Dr P. L. Morosini
Istituto Superiore di Sanità
Laboratorio di Epidemiologia e
Biostatistica
Viale Regina Elena 299
00161 Roma-Nomentano
Italy

Professor Christian Müller
Hôpital de Cery
Clinique Psychiatrique Universitaire
Canton de Vaud
1008 Prilly
Switzerland

Professor Rolf Öhmann
Department of Psychiatry
University Hospital
S-221 85 Lund
Sweden

Professor Carlo Perris
Department of Psychiatry &
WHO Collaborating Center for
Research & Training in Psychiatry,
Umeå University
S-901 85 Umeå
Sweden

Professor R. G. Priest
Academic Department of Psychiatry
St. Mary's Hospital
Praed Street
London W2 1NY
United Kingdom

Professor Ole J. Rafaelsen
Psychochemistry Institute
University Hospital
9, Blegdamsvej
DK-2100 Copenhagen Ø
Denmark

Professor Nils Retterstøl
University of Oslo
Gaustad Hospital
Gaustad
Oslo 3
Norway

Dr Raymond Sadoun
Research Director
National Institute of
Health and Medical Research
INSERM U 110
2ter. Rue d'Alésia
75014 Paris 14
France

Professor E. A. Sand
Ecole de Santé Publique
Campus Erasme
Route de Lennick 808
1070 Bruxelles
Belgium

Professor Erik Strömgren
Institute of Psychiatric Demography
Psychiatric Hospital
DK-8240 Risskov
Denmark

Professor Eugenio Torre
Istituto di Scienze Sanitarie Applicate
dell'Università di Pavia
Cattedra di Igiene Mentale,
via Taramelli 3 A
27100 Pavia
Italy

Professor Per Vaglum
Psychiatric Department 6 B
University of Oslo
Ullevål Hospital
Oslo 1
Norway

Dr Per Vestergaard
Psychiatric Hospital
Aarhus University Institute of
Psychiatry,
DK-8240 Risskov
Denmark

Dr Dermot Walsh
The Medico-Social Research Board
73 Lower Baggot Street
Dublin 2
Ireland

Professor Tómas Helgason
Landspítalinn
National University Hospital
Department of Psychiatry
101 Reykjavík
Iceland

EMRC Secretary:
Dr Erik Schenk
European Science Foundation
1, Quai Lezay Marnésia
F-67000 Strasbourg
France

INTRODUCTION

Introduction

T. HELGASON

In this volume are assembled the papers presented at the second workshop arranged by the Study Group on Mental Illness Research of the European Medical Research Councils (EMRC). EMRC is an association of organizations supporting medical and biomedical research in 14 European countries, which started informal collaboration in 1971 but, 4 years later, was transformed into a Standing Committee of the European Science Foundation.

The aims of the EMRC are to exchange information on science policies and research activities and to identify areas where international cooperation and collaboration are of importance. Research on mental illness is one of the special areas which have been on its agenda for a considerable time. In 1978 the Study Group on Mental Illness Research was set up in order to promote European collaboration in this field. The emphasis is on research on treatment and on the evaluation of treatment. Consequently, the first priorities which engaged the attention of the Study Group can be seen in the title of the first workshop (*Methodology in Evaluation of Psychiatric Treatment*, edited by T. Helgason published by Cambridge University Press in 1983) and again in the title of this workshop.

The study group which planned the second workshop was composed of the editors of the present volume. During the preparation of this report our much cherished member, Professor B. Cronholm, died in October 1983. His knowledge of and experience in psychiatric research as well as his enthusiasm for better treatment and care of psychiatric patients was invaluable in selecting the topics of the EMRC workshop for promoting psychiatric research.

During the past three decades, a major change has taken place in the care and treatment of psychiatric patients, the main breakthrough being the development of effective drugs for treating the major psychoses. A number of psychotherapeutic treatments have also evolved during this period. The burgeoning of new treatments filled mental health workers with optimism, which culminated in the community mental health movement and almost in the belief that it was possible to treat and cure all mental illness, thus making the psychiatric hospital obsolete. Although the optimism has receded somewhat, as exemplified by the identification of the so-called new chronic patient, the development of community care has been carried out to its extreme in Italy, where it was decided to close all psychiatric hospitals and minimize hospital treatment of psychiatric patients. In the light of this, the study group suggested to EMRC that the workshop should be held in Italy and the EMRC in turn approached the CNR (Consiglio Nazionale delle Ricerche) which kindly agreed to act as host.

The aim of all our efforts is to prevent or cure mental illness and, failing that, to improve the quality of our patients' lives as much as possible. Quality of life of the chronic patient has always been a major concern of health personnel. Society at large, however, has always been reluctant to put aside sufficient resources for this purpose. Thus mental hospitals have been allowed to become overcrowded, oversized, and dilapidated – the paradoxical effect of which has been to produce the social breakdown syndrome. This syndrome is in no way confined to patients in psychiatric hospitals as it may develop in other patients and even in non-patients who have to submit to the routine of large institutions such as nursing homes and old-age homes.

In order to counteract the possible ill effects of overcrowded and oversized hospitals, mental health personnel and others have introduced changes, innovations and alternatives to hospital care, especially for those in need of long-term treatment. This has led to the deinstitutionalization of a large number of patients, or should we rather say dehospitalization, as the patients have moved from the hospitals to other types of institution or organization. It is well known that a great number of these patients remain disabled, suffer from residual symptoms, have limited social relations and experience difficulties in finding living quarters or employment. It is thus obvious that the practical conditions of their lives are far worse than those of the population at large. But how do these chronic patients perceive their lives and what life conditions are associated with satisfaction and dissatisfaction within various areas of life? How does their life satisfaction compare with that of the general public, and finally, how does it compare with their own earlier experience? And, most important, how can their quality of life be improved?

In spite of much research there are still major lacunae in the present knowledge which prevent these questions from being answered. The objectives of this volume are to identify problems, ask questions, and discuss methods relevant for new research projects, national or international, related to the topic of the workshop.

The volume is somewhat arbitrarily divided into three main parts: the organizational aspects, the patient aspects, and the public health aspects of needed areas of research on long-term treatment of functional psychoses. There is, of course, some overlap between each of the three themes.

In order to sharpen our research tools as well as our clinical acumen it is necessary to refine and standardize the classification of the phenomena with which we are dealing. A better and more precise diagnostic classification is of great importance in the development and evaluation of treatment. It is also an absolute prerequisite in the effective communication of research results. This is discussed in the first chapter by Strömgren. Besides this chapter, Part I includes chapters on structural changes in hospitals and on alternatives to hospitals as well as chapters on the effects of closing mental hospitals, on further developments in Italy, and on the optimal duration of treatment. Part II comprises chapters dealing with research questions related to different therapeutic methods, psychotherapeutic as well as pharmacological, and rehabilitation. In Part III, the use of case registers in research is discussed, as is research into chronic disability, patient neglect and suicides. The last three papers of the volume deal with research into interaction within families, cost-effectiveness studies and European aspects of the consumption of services.

As it is the purpose of EMRC to identify needed areas of research in medicine and stimulate international research activities, this volume is presented in the hope that the questions it raises will be taken up for further research by the readers. Thus the long-term treatment of functional psychoses will become better, the patients' disability reduced and their quality of life improved.

The study group wants to acknowledge the support and interest of the member councils of EMRC. The active participation of the Chairman of EMRC, Professor H. Danielsson, was of crucial importance in the preparation of the workshop. The assistance of the European Science Foundation and its staff was indispensable and is highly appreciated, special thanks are due to the authors of the chapters in the volume.

Reykjavík, June 1984 Tómas Helgason

I: ORGANISATIONAL ASPECTS OF LONG-TERM TREATMENT

Classification of functional psychoses requiring long-term treatment

E. STRÖMGREN

At first glance it might not seem necessary to provide a special classification of the functional psychoses under study. Such psychoses will have their natural place in current psychiatric classifications, primarily the World Health Organization's (WHO) International Classification of Diseases. Such classifications do not, however, pay special attention to the criteria relating to the need for long-term treatment. It is also obvious that current classifications were originally constructed to serve as the basis for statistics, especially for annual reports of psychiatric institutions. Their focus is therefore mainly on such psychiatric disorders which lead to admission to hospital. In the present study, we are interested not only in cases such as these, but equally in psychotic patients who are treated on an outpatient basis or even are not treated at all. Especially among the latter groups there are disorders which are not easily placed within the official classifications. So for our purpose it may be desirable to make some additions to, and modifications of, official classifications.

The organizers of this workshop have selected for discussion the treatment of functional *psychoses*. They were right to do so since the psychoses are the most incapacitating of all mental disorders. A psychosis changes the identity of the patient's personality, and it is the most urgent responsibility of the psychiatrist to restore the original personality. In addition, choice and maintenance of the right therapy is more important for psychotics than for any other group of the mentally ill. In many cases treatment of psychoses is successful despite the limited facilities and manpower available. It may therefore be regarded as good economy to invest existing resources mainly in the treatment of psychoses (including preventive measures during non-psychotic stages).

Among the psychoses, those which can be called '*functional*' are a special subject of discussion. Although it is quite difficult to define strictly what should be meant by the term, everybody knows, by and large, what is involved. 'Functional' is mostly used in contrast to 'organic' and could therefore logically be substituted by the term 'non-organic'. This seems, however, too daring since it is quite possible that some of the 'functional' psychoses also have an organic basis which is at present unknown, or only vaguely mooted. Among psychoses there are some with known aetiology, some without. Among the latter, the functional psychoses represent the great majority.

Exclusion of the organic psychoses from discussion has the consequence that a great part of gerontopsychiatry will be left out. It should, however, never be forgotten that many psychoses affecting the elderly are of a functional nature. Unfortunately, such psychoses are often regarded as just signs of involution, and they are therefore not treated adequately. Some of the sufferers recover spontaneously, but for many the course of their illness depends on the right diagnosis and the right therapy. In a lot of geriatric institutions there are patients who are treated simply as nursing cases in spite of the fact that therapy might lead to complete recovery. Many similar patients are never admitted to institutions but are in the community and just regarded as geriatric cases.

It is necessary that we acquire information about all relevant cases, regardless of their present location. Countries which are culturally similar may present striking differences with regard to the use of psychiatric institutions. In the WHO publication entitled *Mental Health Services in Europe* (WHO, 1976) this is illustrated in a spectacular way. The number of beds for psychiatric patients per 1000 population varies between 0.2 and 4.6. Even the neighbouring Scandinavian countries show remarkable differences: Denmark 2.3, Norway 2.6, Sweden 3.5, Finland 4.4. Since the incidence and prevalence of mental disorders seem to be practically the same in these countries, one must conclude that the numbers of mentally ill patients treated outside institutions or not treated at all must differ greatly. One of the most urgent tasks must be to find out, by means of epidemiological studies, how many functional psychotics there are, where they are, and whether they receive adequate treatment.

Now to the question of *classification*. Although most psychiatrists feel that diagnostic classification is desirable before well-indicated therapy can be established, others seem to feel that classification is neither useful nor possible. It must be admitted that psychiatric diagnosis has become a more difficult procedure in recent years. So many patients have been treated by all kinds of pharmacotherapy before they reach the psychiatrists that very little of the original symptomatological picture may be left. In a sense we have, to a certain degree, come back to experiencing psychoses as something like the *Einheitspsychose* which was a popular concept in the middle of the nineteenth century. Nowadays we have what could be called the 'pharmacogenic unity psychosis', or maybe the 'comprehensive psychosis', or the 'all-round psychosis'. We have far too many patients who have started with a psychosis the nature of which is no longer clear; these patients have been freely treated with drugs, sometimes regardless of the fact that the psychosis may have been of a short-lasting nature. The patient is then left in a state which may be mainly characterized by drug effects, the therapy being continued simply for prophylactic reasons. This is a disturbing side effect which should not prevent us from doing our best to make a diagnosis as early as possible and to direct therapy accordingly.

The natural starting point for a classification is the International Classification of Diseases (ICD). Here the functional psychoses occupy numbers 295 to 298. The general description of group 295 (schizophrenic psychoses) will probably be accepted by the great majority of psychiatrists. The group is then divided into several subgroups; some of these subgroups are not universally accepted as belonging to schizophrenia. Some are not easily distinguished from each other: simple type, hebephrenic type, latent schizophrenia, residual schizophrenia, and may simply correspond to the 'unity psychoses'.

Subgroup 295.4 (acute schizophrenic episode) will, by many psychiatrists, not be regarded as belonging to schizophrenia. It is my impression that Professor Pichot would be inclined to place the *Bouffées délirantes* here and not, as stated in the ICD, under 298.3 (acute paranoid reaction).

There will be still more disagreement concerning 295.7 (schizoaffective type). Some psychiatrists regard this type as a disorder *per se*; others feel that most of the cases belong to the manic-depressive disorders with which they share the course and the response to treatment. For the purpose of the study of psychoses requiring long-term treatment these differences are, however, of minor importance since the great majority of patients with schizoaffective psychoses are prone to relapse and therefore are often under continuous or frequent treatment over a long period. To a lesser degree this also applies to 'acute schizophrenic episode' and *Bouffées délirantes*; even if the psychotic states are brief, these patients usually have weak and vulnerable personalities and need competent supervision in order to prevent or treat relapses. So there is no doubt that all psychoses included in 295, the schizophrenic psychoses, come within the topic of our workshop.

The situation is similar with 296, the 'affective psychoses'. The clinical description of the different groups does not comply too well with current thinking in continental Europe. In addition, it is questionable whether the types described include all depressive states which are relevant to our topic. It seems, for instance, quite likely that some cases which probably will be placed under 300.4 (neurotic depression) in fact belong to the manic-depressive group even if they are 'pseudoneurotic' in style. They may be mild forms of endogenous affective psychoses and they should be treated as such, often needing long-term prophylactic treatment. Such cases are not very often seen in psychiatric departments and hospitals, but field studies have shown them to be quite common in the community. This was an early experience within the framework of the community mental health project carried out on the Danish island of Samsø since 1957. These patients, who had never been admitted to hospital and had mostly not been treated at all, displayed mild but definite symptoms of endogenous depression; they responded excellently to antidepressant therapy by means of drugs or electroconvulsive therapy (ECT).

I should like to mention also a very recent study by a Danish psychiatrist done in collaboration with a general practitioner (Vanggaard & Jørgensen, 1981). Within a rural general practice of about 3000 inhabitants, the general practitioner had diagnosed 118 cases of depression which he had treated with clomipramine, with remarkable success. These patients were then examined by a very experienced psychiatrist (with special expertise in psychotherapy), who found that 105 of these patients were in fact suffering from endogenous depression. In 75 patients the results of the clomipramine treatment was excellent, in 20 moderately good; 10 patients did not complete the treatment. These results are unusual; the incidence of endogenous depression seems exceptionally high in spite of the fact that the population is probably fairly representative of the Danish non-metropolitan population. But in any case the patients have been in need of treatment, and have profited from it. So this large, non-hospitalized group certainly deserves the serious attention of psychiatrists (Nielsen *et al.*, 1981).

Similar observations concerning high incidence of endogenous depression have, over time, been made in several countries, including Denmark (Lange, 1886), Germany (Bonhoeffer, 1912), and the USA (Campbell, 1953).

ICD's group 297 (paranoid states) is heterogeneous, but all the subgroups contain cases which have long duration and need continued treatment. It is important to stress this point concerning 297.2 (paraphrenia) since these patients are often placed in non-psychiatric institutions, or live on their own and are therefore often not treated at all.

'Other non-organic psychoses' (ICD's group 298) should, according to the glossary to ICD 9, 'be restricted to the small group of psychotic conditions that are largely or entirely attributable to a recent life experience'. Many psychiatrists would say that such psychotic conditions are not at all infrequent. Since these patients have often vulnerable personalities and are living in stressful surroundings, they need continuous support, one of the aims of which is to prevent psychotic relapses. So even if these reactive psychoses are by definition short-lasting, the patients in these cases require long-term treatment.

Here again the glossary blurs the distinction between endogenous and reactive depressions, a distinction which may be of decisive importance for instituting the right therapy.

The different kinds of paranoid psychoses described under group 298 all arise on the basis of vulnerable personality and, even if the paranoid state may be of short duration, the patients need long-term treatment.

In conclusion, I would like to stress that the concept of 'functional psychoses requiring long-term treatment' does certainly not only apply to schizophrenia but also to the majority of endogenous and reactive affective psychoses and paranoid states. There is no doubt that the last two groups are in need of much more therapeutic manpower than the schizophrenic group.

It is conventional to think of psychiatric hospitals as having beds for two different kinds of patients: those who stay for a short time, and those who stay for a long time (frequently becoming chronic inmates). There is indeed a third group which is perhaps the most important: those patients who have psychoses which, in principle, are benign and highly accessible to treatment but who may for a period of years have frequent relapses. During such years these patients need practically continuous support; this support is essential to their whole future since in part it aims to optimize their familial and social relations, even during the possibly long periods when they are obliged to stay in hospital. If these contacts are not preserved, even if after some years the patients recover completely, they may become drop-outs from society.

It goes without saying that also after the years spent mainly in hospital these patients need continuous support and also supervision of preventive treatment. On the whole it looks as if this group of patients with functional psychoses is the one which should occupy the most intensive attention of the mental health services, for the sake of the patients and of society as well.

References

Bonhoeffer, K. (1912). Zur Differentialdiagnose der Neurasthenie und der endogenen Depressionen. *Berliner klinische Wochenschrift*, **29**, 1–4.

Campbell, J. D. (1953). *Manic-depressive Disease*. Philadelphia, London & Montreal: Lippincott Company.

Lange, C. (1886). *Om periodiske Depressionstilstande og deres Patogenese* (*On Periodic Depressions and their Pathogenesis*). Copenhagen: Jacob Lunds Forlag.

Nielsen, J., Nielsen, J. A., Kastrup, M. & Strömgren, E. (eds) (1981). *The Samsø Project*. Aarhus: Aarhus University.

Vanggaard, T. & Jørgensen, B. (1981). Atypiske endogene depressioner i almenpraksis. (Atypical endogenous depressions in general practice). *Månedsskrift for praktisk lægegerning*, **59**, 137–56.

WHO Offset Publication No. 23: May, A. R. (1976). *Mental Health Services in Europe: A Review of Data Collected in Response to a WHO Questionnaire*. Geneva: WHO.

Structural changes in psychiatric hospitals

N. RETTERSTØL

Introduction

In this paper the national situation regarding psychiatric hospital services in Norway, developments during the last 30 years and the 1979 census are presented. Analysis of the Norwegian census throws light on the question of whether there will be a need for psychiatric hospitals in the future.

I will also discuss how psychiatric hospitals can be developed and modernized in their treatment procedures, and how such development is seen by patients and staff. Experiences of structural changes in two Norwegian psychiatric hospitals will be detailed; these point to needed areas of research in this field.

Psychiatric hospitals in Norway – a survey and a census

Great changes have taken place in the structure of psychiatric hospitals. As in most western nations, the ideology shaping mental care in Norway has shifted since World War II from a traditional institutional approach to a community-based concept of treatment for the chronic patient. There is a tendency towards deinstitutionalization. The author will give a report on the 1979 census of mental patients in Norway; this has recently been presented by Øgar (1983) and showed that about half of the mental hospital patients could be expected to remain there because adequate community facilities did not exist.

Until World War II, the 20 mental hospitals formed the cornerstone of care for the chronic mentally ill in Norway, a country of 4000000 inhabitants. Some government statistics illustrate the trend in mental hospital use since the War.

While there has been a reduction in the number of beds since 1964 (Table 1), there has been a marked rise in the number of admissions, especially

Table 1. *In-patients and admission in psychiatric hospitals in Norway 1950–82*

	Number of patients	Admissions
1950	6320	2904
1964	8164	6567
1979	6140	10520
1982	5900	11500

readmissions; this is an indication of more active treatment and rehabilitation efforts. This trend began even before the introduction of neuroleptics, as pointed out by Ødegård (1971).

The diagnostic distribution of patients has changed over the past 30 years. The annual number of first admissions for functional psychoses has been stable at approximately 1000. However, the number for senile and organic psychoses has nearly doubled over the last 20 years, partly due to the increase in longevity. The number of patients suffering from drug or alcohol abuse has increased. Neurotics today represent one third of the admissions to mental hospitals, although they represent only 12% of the resident population of the mental hospitals. They now make up the largest group of first-admission patients. This finding mainly reflects the changing function of the mental hospital, which today has more comprehensive responsibility for psychiatric services within the catchment area, as pointed out by Øgar (1983). The mental hospital is on its way from being isolated and remote to becoming an active insititution with responsibility for the psychiatric services within a catchment area. The number of patients in private care (which was earlier an alternative to mental hospital for chronic psychiatric patients) has, in the same period, fallen from 6000 in 1950 to 1800 in 1978 (Ugelstad, 1978).

In recent years there has been a decrease in the number of long-term mental patients, from 4.5 per 1000 inhabitants in 1955 to 3.2 in 1975 (private care and nursing homes included) (Øgar, 1983).

Those suffering from *functional psychoses* made up the majority of the patients, as seen in Table 2, which also demonstrates the diagnostic composition of the patients in mental hospitals. Long-term patients (those in treatment for 1 year or more) were mostly psychotic; more men than women were diagnosed as suffering from schizophrenia, and more women than men were affected by senile or organic psychoses.

Table 2. *Diagnosis for patients in mental hospitals*

Diagnosis	Frequency[a]	
Functional psychoses		
Schizophrenia	47	64
Affective psychoses	7	
Reactive psychoses etc.	10	
Senile and presenile psychoses	11	
Other organic psychoses	5	
Neuroses	10	
Alcoholism and drug dependence	2	
Character disorders	4	
Other	4	

Note: [a] Figures expressed as a percentage; $N = 6278$.

The long-stay patients were older and had more need for social and practical support than did the short-stay group; the short-stay group had much in common with patients seen in psychiatric departments and clinics. Short-stay patients make up 80% of annual admissions to mental hospitals.

Of the patients in mental hospitals, 62% had been admitted involuntarily, and 49% of those were retained under the Mental Health Act. Those retained against their will had to meet certain criteria in addition to a diagnosis of psychosis. 9% were judged to be dangerous to themselves, 7% dangerous to others. It was thought that recovery would be impaired by discharge in 26% of the cases and that the patient would suffer hardship if discharged in 82%. Only 25% of all the patients were judged to have access to an equal treatment facility outside the hospital, and have a probable gain from being discharged.

From Table 2 it can be seen that the majority of patients now in need of mental hospital facilities belong to the group of functional psychoses. The results of the nation-wide census (Øgar, 1983), taken of all mental patients under care, particularly long-term patients, in November 1979 include the figures for patients under care (Table 3).

As a whole, the patients in general hospital psychiatric departments were quite different from the other institutionalized ill; they were younger and 63% were women. They represented mainly short-term patients with fairly good contact with family and work, though 25% were diagnosed as having a functional psychosis. The patients in psychiatric nursing homes presented

Table 3. *Census November 1979*

	Number of patients
In psychiatric hospitals	6278
In psychiatric nursing homes	4058
In psychiatric departments (in general hospitals)	992
In psychiatric half-way houses	188
In psychiatric private care	526
Total	12042

the other extreme; 75% were more than 60 years old, 85% had been in institutions for more than 1 year, and 26% for more than 10 years. A large proportion needed considerable nursing care.

The patients in psychiatric hospitals presented an intermediate picture: about evenly divided between men and women; most (38%) were aged 50–69 years; a large proportion (27%) were aged 70 years or more; 65% were aged over 50 years; 60% were unmarried, 22% were widowed or divorced; only 18% were married. However, there is also a big group of patients belonging to the diagnostic group of senile, presenile and other organic psychoses. There is, therefore, clearly a strong need for differentiation of the treatment facilities.

The great reduction of the number of in-patients has been possible due to several circumstances, of which the most important seems to be the more active therapeutic procedures within the hospitals (included milieu-therapy), a more active discharge policy, better out-patient facilities and after-care arrangements.

Was the stay in mental hospital necessary for the patients, or could they have been treated outside hospital?

The research group in the nationwide census evaluated the material carefully to determine what placement and work or other activity would be most appropriate for the 6278 hospitalized patients, and what placement or activity they realistically could expect to receive (Øgar, 1983). Only 1074 patients (less than 20%) were found to be appropriate candidates for continued hospitalization. However, realistically 3050 could be expected to remain in the hospital; this left around 2000 who were inappropriately placed because of a lack of suitable alternatives.

The researchers applied the same method to all 12042 patients in all facilities and found that a total of 1301 new alternative placements were needed (517 in psychiatric nursing homes, 228 in psychiatric day hospitals, 289 in half-way houses and 267 in group sheltered homes). Moreover, they identified a need for 1100 new residential placements, 543 sheltered work placements and 273 ordinary jobs outside the psychiatric services. Most of the placements were needed for long-term patients with functional psychoses. Other countries have reported similar problems in finding appropriate placements for patients (Report on a Working Group, WHO, 1978). It can be concluded that we need the psychiatric hospitals, but they can be reduced to fewer, smaller and more effective institutions if suitable alternatives are built up.

There is need for further research along these lines within the same country at certain intervals in order to evaluate the development. The evaluation will of course change as the social pattern outside changes (for instance, with increasing or decreasing unemployment). Research along these lines should also be stimulated in other countries.

Structural changes and their evaluation

During the last 20 years great changes have taken place in the psychiatric hospitals, which have made development possible. However, structural changes have to be initiated and evaluated.

When I took over the male department, Gaustad Hospital, 1 January 1973, I used the valuable experience of reconstruction of a traditional psychiatric hospital gained during the 4 years of my leadership of the psychiatric hospital in Bergen. This reconstruction has been described (Retterstøl, 1974) and evaluated (Ose, 1976). The evaluation was done 4 years after the structural changes were started and, therefore, gave only limited feed-back on the restructuring of treatment procedures.

Planning the evaluation

At the very beginning of the structural changes (actually before they started) I applied for a research worker whose task would be the evaluation of the development. This was granted. The question then arose regarding the background of the evaluator. Should it be a sociologist who could be an observer from outside, or should it be a psychiatrist, familiar with work and life in a psychiatric hospital? We chose the latter, partly because he could be seen by the patients as a helper and also because he could be given limited clinical tasks. The researcher worked out his own instruments and used his own tools, as described (Waal, 1978).

The structural changes

These were developed gradually, much emphasis being laid on informing all the staff groups and also taking their ideas into consideration. The structural changes have been described in detail (Retterstøl, 1979). The central reforms included a gradual stepping down of the hierarchical structure, increased decentralization at ward level and an increase in the number of more qualified staff members responsible for the psychotherapy and milieu-therapy. Over 4 years, the number of doctors doubled (13 to 26), the number of psychologists trebled (from 2 to 6) and the number of social workers quadrupled (from 2 to 8). Intensified group and milieu-therapy was started in one of the wards and was gradually introduced into other wards. Out-patient facilities, which had up to then been non-existent, were started (including pre-care and after-care). A school was established; during the first years it increased its number of teachers from 1 to 6 and is still expanding. A special service was started for the treatment of young drug dependents. A training programme was initiated for the staff (including the nurse aids). Particular mention should be made of a small ward (6–8 patients) for young schizophrenic patients in danger of chronification. Gradually, young schizophrenic patients in the hospital system got the opportunity of having 1 year's treatment in this ward. After some years it was seen that 1 year was too short a period; we now give 2 years of intensive treatment. The development of this pioneer ward has been described by Ugelstad (1978) and Haugsgjerd (1983).

The evaluation

Waal, utilized a systematic theoretical line of thought and nomenclature in his study, and his findings are also presented in separate reports (Waal, 1976, 1977). He analysed the general development and the various meetings through personal attendance and through interviews and questionnaire-based investigations among participants. By this means, there soon appeared signals to the management about unfortunate trends that could be corrected at an early stage. He showed clearly that the way from a simple hierarchical to an open structure is a complicated process. But he also demonstrated that the increased democratization paved the way for greater active participation and well-being among large groups of the staff.

Furthermore, analyses of milieu-therapy revealed that there was a need for more differentiated wards than had been developed. It also became evident that the introduction of milieu therapy in a department called for the injection of personnel. Another finding was a marked increase in the circulation of voluntary patients wishing to attend the more attractive therapeutic offers. The proportion of voluntary patients rose from 50% in 1969 to 80% in 1976. During the years 1973 to 1976 the number of in-patients was reduced to two-thirds and the number of admissions doubled.

On the other hand, analysis of the total patient population showed that, in the doctors' opinion, only 19% of the patients were in need of active therapeutic measures (according to the nurses this applied to only 15%, according to the patients only 7%). In other words, intensive therapeutic measures were indicated in a limited number of wards.

The requirement for good nursing was the principal reason for a continued stay; in the doctors' view this applied to 46%, in the staffs' view to 38%, and in the patients' view to 29%. These experiences from our hospital are in good accordance with the findings of Øgar (1982) in a nationwide investigation of the patients in psychiatric hospitals, where he estimated about two-thirds of the patients to be mainly in need of care. Therefore, active milieu-therapy of a more psychotherapeutic approach is suitable for only a limited number of patients in psychiatric hospitals – it may be useful in some wards, harmful in others and of no sense in many. In Norway, Friis (1981) has in several studies pointed to the importance of differentiating the wards as to the functional levels of the patients and activity, using standardized methods as WAS (Ward Atmosphere Scale).

Degree of satisfaction with the structural changes within the different occupational groups was assessed by means of systematic interviews and forms. The doctors all experienced the development as positive and found their work absorbing and interesting. None of them wished to return to the hierarchial structure. But the working stress had increased; meetings, in particular, took up much time. This also applied for the psychologists and social workers.

The vast majority of the trained nursing staff expressed satisfaction with the changes. They felt that their occupational group was in the thick of things, and that their status had risen (not least in eyes of the doctors). They had acquired more responsibility and independence, and thought they were the group most positively affected by the structural changes. The assistant nurses also reacted favourably.

The group of 'old nursing aids' was the most sceptical, especially of group- and milieu-therapy. A common complaint was that the development had passed them by, and they felt that their work was not sufficiently appreciated. The group was, however, stable and loyal, found cooperation good, and thought the reconstruction had been beneficial for the patients. However, the reaction clearly shows that the nursing wards – in which most of them were working – had been overlooked in the general change for the better. The result of this finding was that more attention was turned to these wards, which in the next run received their share of resources.

Those working on the night shift expressed dissatisfaction; this is not surprising taking into consideration that the new methods seldom reached those working at night. To make up for this, a training programme was set up for them. From time to time conflicts arose between the day and night teams. 'Clarification rounds' proved helpful in such instances.

The patients' view was more difficult to assess; there are many methodological problems in the assessment of a patient's conception of his/her treatment and hospital stay. Patients with a passive, dependent personality structure may be expected to respond positively in an effort to please the authorities. Aggressive, immature patients in permanent opposition to authority may be expected to answer negatively. Senile and deteriorated patients are often unable to form an opinion at all.

Waal used two approaches in order to estimate the patients' viewpoints. One approach was a questionnaire in which the patients were asked whether they had noticed any change during the previous 2 years and, if so, whether these had been for the better or for worse. Of the patients who answered and who had been in the hospital long enough to have experienced the change, 82% (of 86 patients) said they had noticed the changes. 65% were of the opinion that the changes were for the better, 15% for the worse. 25% found conditions vastly improved, whereas 42% thought the improvement moderate.

Thus, taken all together, the reception was a favourable one. The most satisfied were patients in the small wards, which had undergone radical structural changes and become more active. When patients were asked whether they wanted further changes, only 16% answered yes. This suggested that others, besides patients, must be responsible for changes. Patients are not a strong pressure group.

The second approach yielded more interesting information. A group of readmitted patients, whose first stay dated from before the structural changes, were interviewed about their impressions of their present and their previous stays. They were also asked about events that had impressed them, their opinion about specific changes, and whether they would recommend the hospital to others with the same troubles as their own. They were promised anonymity. The interviewer was not directly associated with the hospital management, nor had he been involved with the reconstruction set-up. The response was almost unanimous that the changes were very positive. Especially appreciated was the relaxation of strict rules, and the greater degree of liberty.

Further research

Isohanni (1983) from the University of Oulu has presented systematized experiences on the psychiatric ward as a therapeutic community, and also discussed the influence of changes on treatment outcomes in a psychiatric ward and the problems of leadership. Leadership is difficult, but crucial for successful results of structural changes. Research on leadership therefore will be an important topic in the future, as will also be the question of which patients will profit from which structural changes in a hospital setting. There can be hardly any doubt that a ward setting fit for one category of patients may be less fruitful, or even harmful for another group. From Norway, research by Friis (1981) and Vaglum (1979) clearly indicates the importance of differentiating the wards in terms of the functional levels of the patients. Refined methods in this field of research are urgently called for.

Conclusion

Areas of research on long-term treatment of functional psychoses for which there is an apparent need are:

1. *Census investigations* at certain intervals (e.g. every fifth year) of patients in mental institutions in a country, or part of it. In such investigations the needs of the individual patient must also be evaluated. Is there a need for further treatment in a psychiatric institution or not? If the answer is not: what would be the best alternative? From census investigations of this kind, the appropriate alternatives can be compiled.
2. *Evaluation of structural changes in psychiatric hospitals* should be stimulated, and possibly even planned before structural changes are initiated. The development within a hospital can profit from a systematic investigation of the consequences of the procedures taken.
3. *Investigations on the structural changes necessary to promote cure or improvement in the conditions of different groups of patients suffering from functional psychoses* should be undertaken.

References

Friis, S. (1981). Hva slags postatmosfære er terapeutisk for psykotiske pasienter? *Tidskrift for den Norske lægeforening*, **101**, 848–85.

Haugsgjerd, S. (1983). *Psykoterapi ved psykoser* (ved psykotiske tilstander). Oslo: Universitetsforlaget.

Isohanni, M. (1983). The psychiatric ward as a therapeutic community. Acta Universitatis Ouluensis, University of Oulu, Finland.

Ose, E. (1976). *Virkninger av Strukturendringer i Psykiatriske Sykehus*. Oslo: Universitetsforlaget.

Report on a Working Group (1978). *Constraints in Mental Health Development.* Copenhagen: W(orld) H(ealth) O(rganization) Regional Office for Europe.

Retterstøl, N. (1974). *Det Psykiatriske Sykehus i Omforming.* Oslo: Universitetsforlaget.

Retterstøl, N. (1979). *Det Psykiatriske Sykehus i Omforming II.* Oslo: Universitetsforlaget.

Ugelstad, E. (1978). *Psykotiske Langtidspasienter i Psykiatriske Sykehus – Nye behandlingsforsøk.* Oslo: Universitetsforlaget.

Vaglum, P. (1979). Unge stoffmisbrutere i et terapeutisk samfunn. Oslo: Universitetsforlaget

Waal, H. (1976). Styringsproblemer i psykiatrien – Situasjonsanalyse ved behandlingsinstitusjonene som et åpent system. *Nordisk Psykiatrisk Tidskrift*, **8**, 609–20.

Waal, H. (1977). Rolleforandringer for leger, psykologer og sosionomer under strukturendringer i det psykiatriske sykehus *Tidskrift for den Norske lægeforening*, **97**, 846–8.

Waal, H. (1978). *Psykiatriske Sykehus – Utviklingsmuligheter og Begrensninger.* Oslo: Universitetsforlaget.

Ødegård, Ø. (1971). Hospitalized Psychoses in Norway: Time Trends 1926–1963. *Social Psychiatry*, **6**, 53–8.

Øgar, B. (1982). *Patients in psychiatric institutions: a census study.* Trondheim: Norwegian Institute of Hospital Research.

Øgar, B. (1983). Recent developments in the care, treatment and rehabilitation of the chronic mentally ill in Norway. *Hospital and Community Psychiatry*, **34**, 348–52.

Alternatives to hospitals: a field of promises and of not-yet answered questions

C. PERRIS

The search for alternatives to hospitals for the care of mentally ill people is a concern shared by the industralized as well as the developing countries. In the former, this arises mainly because of the criticism of mental institutions that has grown stronger and stronger during the last decades. In the latter, it is because the organization of psychiatric care is still in its infancy and a policy must be chosen whether to utilize scarce resources in an attempt to build up an appropriate network of hospitals (and for which patients), or whether other, less expensive alternatives should be favoured. These might enable similar therapeutic goals to be reached. Since developing countries do not yet have the potential to carry out thorough evaluation projects, it might be assumed that they look at what is planned in the industrialized world in a search for guidelines to follow in their own planning. Thus, our responsibility in advocating different alternatives for the care of the mentally ill might have a much wider implication than would be assumed at first glance.

Finding alternatives to hospitals seems to be a major issue for policy makers, psychiatrists, and pressure groups of different kinds. The argument for less institutional care has often been put in a boasting, rhetorical way (and has appeared, sometimes, to be a goal in itself). Also, it is not always clear whether such a stress on alternatives is based on a common rationale or whether this apparently common goal conceals disparate values and interests. In view of a certain difficulty in disentangling different objectives, I feel that 'alternatives to hospitals' cannot be discussed in a meaningful way unless additional basic concepts are taken into account. In fact, before discussing alternatives, and eventially advocating any of their possible advantages, it is necessary to establish:

1. which kind of hospital could (or should) be substituted and
2. which kind of patient is referred to.

In addition to the above-mentioned issues, it is essential to consider the broader sociocultural context. By 'sociocultural context' I mean primarily such variables as the economic level of the country, and the level of development and comprehensiveness of systems of general health and social care. In addition variables such as values, attitudes, and level of education in the general population (which are more difficult to measure) should also be given serious consideration.

Hospitals to which alternatives are sought

Although the provision of shelter and care for the mentally ill was practised long before the beginning of the Christian era, the movement that eventually led to the widespread establishment of the traditional mental hospital as understood today did not really start until after the social transformation brought about the French Revolution. Both the idea of liberating people from bondage, and a religious revival were essential to further the humanistic efforts of the supporters of the mental hospital movement in the first half of the nineteenth century. Dorothea Dix, the social reformer, was one of the first to initiate the hospital movement; she strongly believed not only in the humanistic character of the institution, but also that it was cheaper to take charge of the insane in a curative institution than to support them for life elsewhere (Deutsch, 1949). Another powerful force that contributed to the establishment of mental institutions was their identification as a mechanism of social control to protect the community from dangerous individuals.

According to Foucault (1965), the institutionalization of the mentally ill was nothing more than an attempt to bring madness under the rigid control of reason. Thus, the rationale that led to the development and establishment of traditional mental hospitals was based on the following three tenets:

1. decentralized mental institutions, away from big urban conglomerates were the most suitable place for the application of the curative principles of 'moral treatment' that had been advocated by such enlightened pioneers as Pinel in France, Tuke in England. and Rush in the USA;
2. mental hospitals could provide moral treatment and have a curative function at a reasonably low cost; and
3. mental hospitals represented a suitable mechanism of social control to mould the insane into something more acceptable to society.

However, in the course of time, the ability of the hospital to justify its existence on the basis of any of these three counts was successively eroded. Increasing admission rates, which very soon led to uncontrollable overcrowding, and a decline in the belief of the curative value of moral treatment, discredited the hospital's 'curative' potential and challenged its suitability to meet humanistic goals at a reasonable expense. Not only that: relatively recent investigations in the late 1950s and early 1960s showed unequivocally that hospital care had changed from curative to custodial, and that its impact on the patient was more detrimental than beneficial (Barton, 1976; Goffman, 1961; Wing, 1962; Gruenberg, 1966). In the period immediately after World War II, it was calculated that if this situation had to be changed substantially (that is, if mental hospitals were to be raised to an acceptable standard with respect to both buildings and manpower), then the cost would be enormous. In the USA, for example, it was estimated that to bring the existing hospitals up to the standard set up by the American Psychiatric Association would require a sum of $4000000000 (Karno & Schwartz, 1974).

The mental hospital's function as a mechanism of social control has been the strongest and most enduring. However, the rise of the Civil Rights movement in the 1960s has challenged this function as well, in view of the abuses perpetrated in its name. Such a challenge has been pushed to such a degree as to cause major modifications in admission and retention procedures in most industrialized countries. In the Italian Reform Law of 1978, for example the concept of 'dangerousness' has been omitted from the indications for commitment.

From what I have written so far, it is clear that a search for alternatives has been primarily understood as a search for alternatives to traditional mental hospitals. In fact, radical decisions have already been made in many Western countries to cope with the problem. Among the early decisions, there has been a drive to bring psychiatry back into a medical context through the implementation of psychiatric departments in general hospitals. Efforts have been directed not only towards obtaining a substantial reversal of the trend in admissions (which had been steadily increasing) but also at phasing out the existing hospitals.

In this context, a new movement emerged characterized by a shift of the focus from care in hospitals to care in the community, with the concept of deinstitutionalization as one of its most important principles. It is very likely that 'deinstitutionalization' was understood at the very beginning as the process of moving those patients from mental hospitals who were kept in custody, but were not actively treated. However, the concept has successively become much broader in its scope. Brown (1975), in his often-quoted definition of deinstitutionalization, takes into account not only the release into the community of all institutional patients, but also the prevention of inappropriate mental hospital admissions through the provision of community-based treatment alternatives. Although Brown explicitly referred to the prevention of 'inappropriate' admissions to 'mental hospitals', this precept has probably been interpreted very widely in many quarters and has been expanded to refer to any kind of admission and to any kind of hospital, including the departments of psychiatry in general hospitals. Most of the debate on the reorganization of psychiatric care that occurred in Sweden in the 1970s was focussed on a shift from in-patient care to care in out-patient units or in day- and night-hospitals independent of the type of hospital where an admission would otherwise have occurred. Apparently, similar to the way in which a strong belief in the curative potential of moral treatment led to the establishment of the mental hospital, a strong belief in the curative potential of psychotherapeutic approaches and of social intervention led to a generalized negation of the appropriateness of in-patient care. However, a closer scrutiny of this more recent process suggests that no adequate attention has been paid to possible differential needs of different categories of patients.

The patients for whom alternatives to hospitals are discussed

One major problem in traditional mental hospitals has been the admission of patients with a wide range of morbid conditions. No doubt, the main reason for admitting many of these was not that they were in need of care at such a mental hospital, but that more appropriate facilities were lacking. Evidence for that can be obtained by comparing the composition of in-patient populations in different countries set against the general organization of care systems. In countries where the care of the mentally retarded developed separately from that of the mentally ill, the proportion of mentally retarded among in-patients at mental hospitals is negligible compared with that in those countries where such an organizational separation does not exist. Variations in this respect occur not only among countries, but also within single countries. In West Germany, for example, the proportion of mentally retarded in mental hospitals has been reported to vary from about 5% to more than 25% in different parts of the country (Deutscher Bundestag, Drucksache 7/4200, 1975). Another factor to be taken into account is the degree of development of geriatric and of long-care services. Where such services are undifferentiated or not developed at all, or where their capacity is far below the real needs of the population, many geriatric and long-care patients will be found in mental hospitals.

Both in the USA and in Britain there has been a pronounced decline

Table 1. *Number of in-patients in the age group 65 years or older present in different American institutions in 1969 and in 1973*

Type of institution	1969	1973
State and county hospitals	111420	70615
Private mental hospitals	2460	1534
Veterans Administration hospitals	9675	5819
Nursing homes	96415	193900
Total	219970	271868

in the mental hospitals' patient population. However, especially in the USA, few of the patients who have left mental hospitals have actually been deinstitutionalized. In fact, for a large proportion of them, the process has been one of transinstitutionalization rather than of deinstitutionalization (Kernberg, 1981). Table 1, adapted from Regier & Taube (1981), illustrates this point as it relates to older patients.

Also calculations made by the NIMH (DEW Publication ADM-77-433) of the distribution of persons in institutions per 100000 population in 1950 and in 1970 in the USA demonstrate that the results presented in Table 1 apply to patients in all age groups.

Obviously, I do not contest that admission to a nursing home or to some other facility should be regarded as a more appropriate alternative to admission to a mental hospital. My point is that there is a substantial difference between maintaining that psychiatric hospitals should not be misused, and maintaining that all kinds of institutional care should be denied. In fact, whereas in the former the development of suitable alternatives becomes a compelling task, in the latter, a reduction in the mental hospital population followed by the eventual closure of the hospitals becomes a goal in itself, without any regard for the prospects of the deinstitutionalized patients. In addition, it has still to be demonstrated that transinstitutionalization really implies an improvement in the quality of patients' life that goes beyond the valued advantage that they are no longer in a mental hospital.

Another group that I would like to mention in this context is that of the alcoholics and drug abusers. Legislation in many countries, for example in Sweden, provides for alternative care facilities for this group of patients. However, many of them are admitted to mental hospitals and often remain there for very long periods. Such was the situation, for example in Italy, where special facilities for inebriates did not exist.

Consequently, when considering alternatives to hospitals, policy makers should decide where these patients are to be treated if they are in need of in-patient care beyond that of a short period at an acute detoxification unit.

Alternatives to hospitals for the long-term care of patients with functional psychoses

The term 'functional psychoses' is no more than one of the many eponyms used to refer to psychopathological conditions for which there is no assumption about an organic causative role. In practice, the term refers to schizophrenic, affective, and reactive psychotic conditions. Since the last two are most frequently of a transient albeit often recurrent nature, concern as to long-term institutional care refers principally to patients suffering from schizophrenic syndromes. Thus, in discussing alternatives to hospitals for patients with functional psychoses, I will refer in the first place to the care of schizophrenic patients. On the other hand, much of what will be said could be applied to the care of other categories of patients suffering from other psychotic conditions which have shown a tendency towards chronicity.

There is a great amount of evidence supporting the view that the level of disability shown by chronic schizophrenic patients is largely determined by different contributing factors. Using the terminology proposed by Wing (in Wing & Hailey, 1972), three types of impairment should be distinguished. First of all, there is the impairment due to the illness itself, e.g. a psychological blunting that remains after acute symptoms have subsided. Then there are secondary impairments characterized by behavioural reactions, which almost invariably occur whenever primary impairments are present. Last, there is an element consisting of handicaps which exist in most psychiatric patients independently of any illness, e.g. lack of occupational or social skills due to poor education (these are more pronounced the earlier the onset of the disorder) or lack of coping ability. Obviously, the ideal goal of psychiatric care would be the elimination of all three types of handicap. However, a more pragmatic goal is that of reducing these disabilities to a minimum which allows the patient to live a satisfactory social life in the community. If so then, in discussing alternatives to mental hospitals, instead of putting the question 'Why alternatives?' one could ask for which of the above-mentioned impairments care in a mental hospital is most appropriate. My guess is that if the question were expressed in this way, the likely answer would be that care in a hospital is not a necessary prerequisite for reducing any of the three types of impairment. On the contrary, there is enough evidence that prolonged institutional care is one of the most powerful factors contributing to the occurrence of secondary handicaps. The concepts of 'institutional neurosis' (Barton, 1976), 'institutionalism' (Wing, 1962), 'social breakdown syndrome' (Gruenberg, 1967) are too well known to require any comment. Also well documented, is the hypothesis that time in hospital is linearly related to the development of institutionalism (Honigfeld & Gillis, 1967; Wing, 1962; Paul, 1969).

That schizophrenic patients in a relatively stable phase of illness can be appropriately cared for in settings other than in hospital is not a recent discovery. In fact, foster care in private homes was one of the most-used alternatives during the first half of the present century both in the USA and in Europe, and especially in the Scandinavian countries (Davis, 1962; Perris, 1966). In the USA, Morrissey (1967) reported that in 1963 there were some 13000 mentally ill people in family-care homes, plus an additional 4000 in programmes operated by the Veterans Administration. In the Swedish county of Västerbotten, where I am working, there were in 1967 about 150 patients in family-care (that is about 15% of the total in-patient population of the county). However, although supervised family-care has had some rehabilitating function in Sweden, and accordingly some turnover, structured programmes to maximize its rehabilitating potential have never been consistently applied, nor has its use been consciously understood as a purposeful means of pursuing deinstitutionalization. Looking at it retrospectively, it is very likely that the development of family-care has been based on two premises: it was less expensive than hospitalization, and it could free beds for acutely ill patients (Lee, 1963). However, Segal & Aviram (1978) point out very aptly, that family-care programmes, and the development of an organization to supervise them have been among the most direct precursors of the establishment of a community-care system, despite their small scale.

The formal development of other alternatives: day- and night-hospitals, half-way houses, boarding houses, group-homes, sheltered workshops, therapeutic communities, former-patient clubs, lodges etc., is of much more recent date even if informal parallels may have existed for a long time. Each of these alternatives has its advocates and, for many of them, very encouraging results have been reported. However, the number of patients who have been involved in these alternatives is still comparatively small, especially for some, and no thorough comparative evaluations have been carried out that would allow the advocacy of any as the most suitable. I do not feel that an analysis of these above-mentioned alternatives would be useful at this juncture. Instead, I prefer to refer to some broader issues which might be more relevant, and which will allow me to go back to what I have written at the beginning of this paper: namely, each alternative can potentially be better or worse than the hospital depending upon the social context in which it is implemented, its real purpose, and the type of resources devoted to it.

The approach to any kind of alternative to hospitals should be pragmatic and devoid of rhetoric. Alternatives to hospitals should not be born only of the necessity to repair earlier errors made by policy makers, as happened in the USA and is happening in Italy. Instead, they should be planned carefully at the very beginning of a process of deinstitutionalization; their function and limits should be correctly identified. Also, in the planning of alternatives, one should not forget that it is for the future, that is beyond the time limits of an initial brief enthusiasm. For each of the chosen alternatives one should be able to set goals and define objectives and suggest what will be the criteria of success. If this is not done, then the risk will exist that patients are moved from the hospital's backyards to several smaller backyards in the community.

I do not believe that the different alternatives that I have mentioned above are interchangeable or that all of them are similarly suitable in every social context, or for any kind of patients. I am only sure, that any of them can result in failure if attention is not paid to the type of patients expected to utilize it, to the social structure of the place where the alternative is planned, to the availability of collateral community services, and to the level of tolerance of deviance of the resident population within which the alternative is implemented. Uncontrolled deinstitutionalization, independent of any chosen alternative, has produced a backlash in the USA and, to some extent, in Italy as well. Evidence of this unwanted negative effect can be found in accounts of the exploitation of deinstitutionalized patients, in the increasing tendency to criminalize deviant behaviour by mentally ill people, and in the helpless protests of relatives' associations. If one of the important functions of the mental hospital in a particular society has been that of a mechanism of social control, then rejecting reactions can be expected in the community, even when alternatives are adequately supervised and smoothly operated.

All too often it is stressed that alternatives are cheaper than care in hospital. Goldberg (this volume) will probably tell us that it is indeed true, at least in the long run. However, I am a little suspicious when heavy stress is put on economical aspects. In fact, there is a risk that policy makers will underestimate the real costs, especially in an initial – and hopefully transitional – phase when both the existing hospitals, and the new alternatives have to be operated simultaneously.

A restructured hospital: is there a place for it in the future psychiatric organization?

Having reached this point, the reader might have wondered why I did not touch upon the issue of whether all kinds of hospital should be dismantled, or whether hospitals have still a place if they are thoroughly restructured. An answer can be sought from different angles. First of all, it would be necessary to establish whether we mean special hospitals, still isolated from the rest of medical care, or whether we refer to any kind of hospital (i.e. also to psychiatric departments in general hospitals which might provide long-term care besides acute treatment). Second, some agreement should be reached on whether we believe that some kind of social control of deviant behaviour determined by mental illness is still required and, if so, how it should be obtained. Third, we should try to analyse whether restructured psychiatric hospitals are really as effective as we expect them to be in facilitating not only the return of the patient to the community but also the patient's survival in the community. Last, we should try to analyse whether there is some other function of the hospital, not yet discussed in the present paper, that we should consider when talking of alternatives.

As to the first point, there seems to be a general consensus that special psychiatric hospitals, isolated from the rest of the community belong to the past, and that they should not have any place in future planning. Less unanimous however, are opinions as to whether psychiatric in-patient services should or should not be an integral part of the rest of medical care. On this point different ideologies compete with each other. In particular, those who oppose a 'medicalization' of psychiatry see the establishment of special psychiatric departments in general hospitals as a major risk. Paradoxically, this fear has been counteracted in some quarters in Italy by preferring to admit patients in need of psychiatric care into common medical wards at general hospitals. In the USA, side by side with the establishment of psychiatric wards in general hospitals, there has been an establishment of Community Mental Health Centers – often with a considerable number of beds – completely separated from the general hospitals.

Departments at general hospitals in some countries are comprised of wards in which patients can be kept for as long as is necessary for them to qualify for the definition of 'long-stay'. In Italy, the law of 1978 prescribed rules for acute diagnostic and therapeutic interventions and stated that such interventions should occur in general hospitals through, or without the implementation of special psychiatric wards. Some time limits were also stated in the law (establishing how long a patient could be kept in hospital). However, the time limit can be prolonged by periods of three months, apparently indefinitely. At present, the patients' length of stay is very short in almost all Italian special psychiatric units. However, it should be kept in mind that the number of beds available in such units is very low and that the pressure for admission is very high (Perris *et al.*, 1983). In Sweden and as far as I know in Britain as well, there is no time limit that regulates the length of stay of voluntary patients at general hospitals. Although the patients' turnover is usually high, patients can occasionally remain in hospital for a long time. According to official programmes (Socialstyrelsen 1980:2; SPRI, 1982), only wards for acute treatment should exist at the general hospitals in Sweden in the near future, whereas rehabilitation should take place in other kinds of specialized wards. Where these wards, or facilities should be located is, however, not clearly stated yet.

In Sweden, Italy, and in many other countries, committed patients can be admitted to wards in general hospitals; the length of their stay is not necessarily longer than that of voluntarily admitted patients. Such a practice, however, is not currently used in the USA where committed patients are, as a rule, referred to special services, often in a mental hospital. Admittedly, there is no risk that a patient admitted to a psychiatric ward of a general hospital will remain in the hospital for tens of years or for his lifetime, as could happen in the old mental hospitals. Furthermore, the quality of care in such departments is decidedly higher, more open, more active and less custodial. However, several investigations (Caffey *et al.*, 1968; Caffey, Galbecht & Klett, 1971; Glick, Hargreawes & Goldfield, 1974; Herz *et al.*, 1977) suggest that length of stay is not a decisive variable in predicting survival in the community after discharge. In fact, in the studies just mentioned, it was found that rates of readmission were similar, independent of the length of the prior hospitalization. However, the total time in the community was longer for the patients who had received a shorter initial treatment. Also there is some evidence suggesting that hospital admission in itself might have a negative effect on the patient's later adjustment in the community (Test & Stein, 1975).

The issue of social control is of too wide a scope to be discussed here in detail. In my opinion, it is very likely, that societies will continue to need such a mechanism in the future. In this regard, I feel that we balance on an edge: a complete lack of social control is likely to lead to a criminalization of the mentally ill as has occurred in the USA (Segel & Aviram, 1978) and to some extent in Italy (Perris *et al.*, 1983). A too broad use of the hospital for a social-control function is likely to lead to an abuse of psychiatry. The major concern of legislators must be the provision of effective mechanisms of protection of the civil rights of the committed patients. The need for a social-control function is closely related to the level of tolerance in the community. However, the concept of tolerance has hardly been discussed so far, despite of the fact that mechanisms of rejection of deinstitutionalized patients have been operating for a while in many quarters (Segal & Aviram, 1978).

The Western World is at present in a phase of economic depression, and the economic resources of many non-Western countries are far below their real needs. Under such circumstances it is highly improbable that most countries will have the means to develop and to test alternatives to hospitals which will have the capacity to deal both with the patient population that already exists in the traditional mental hospitals, and with the new generations of patients which tend to accumulate. Thus, existing hospitals will probably still be needed, at least in the near future and for some categories of patients. Nevertheless, their structure must change radically.

Admittedly, not all mental hospitals of our time are 'snake pits' practising a dehumanizing custodial care. On the contrary, many of them have evolved towards a very high standard, characterized by a more democratic and open atmosphere, better staff–patient ratios, and innovative treatment and after-care programmes, both in the USA (Gottesfeld, 1977) and in Europe (Jones, 1972; Retterstøl, 1974; Astrup, Dahl & Retterstøl, 1980; Helgason, 1982). However, efforts at making in-hospital treatment more effective seem to have produced relatively disappointing results, especially with the category of patients on which this volume has focussed. In fact, several studies suggest that while intensive-treatment programmes are effective in improving within-hospital adjustment and increasing release rates, it appears that within-hospital adjustment is only in part related to post-hospital adjustment, and is not the least related to length of survival in the community (Fairweather, 1964; Paul, 1969).

There are some other functional aspects of the hospitals which I have not touched upon so far, which must be taken into account when thinking of alternatives. In concluding this chapter, I should like to mention some of them in an indirect way, as questions which need to be answered.

1. To what extent will the abolition of the hospitals lead to an exploitation of the mentally ill, and how can this be counteracted?
2. To what extent will the use of alternatives to hospitals (for example the practise of partial hospitalization) represent such a burden on the patients' families as to lead to a future increase of people with mental problems?

3. Since mental hospitals have been the place where the training of staff has occurred, how should the staff be retrained to be effective in other settings, and how should the training of future staff be organized?
4. If the hospital was a main place for local employment how can we counteract the fear that its closing down will lead to increased unemployment?

Conclusions

I have presented in this paper some of the major issues which should be considered in a meaningful discussion of alternatives to hospitals and pointed out some of the questions that should be answered. My personal opinion is that in-patient treatment might still be regarded as one appropriate alternative for the acute treatment of patients with functional psychoses, although other alternatives in other settings might prove to be as effective if carefully planned. It is also my opinion, that pure in-patient care is not the most appropriate alternative for the habilitation or rehabilitation of patients who have gone through an acute episode. Even if such rehabilitation is hospital-based, much of the work should occur directly in the community. Long-term treatment does not need a hospital setting either in re-structured old mental hospitals or in modern wards at general hospitals. To avoid this kind of hospitalization several alternatives have been proposed, and still others could be developed.

We do not know which alternative, if any, is the one that should consistently be preferred. It is likely, that different alternatives will prove to be most suitable in different places depending upon the social context in which they will be developed. It is also my opinion that the development of alternatives should be planned well in advance before any restriction of the use of the hospitals is implemented. In doing this planning, attention should be paid not only to short-term effects, but also to long-term consequences.

References

Astrup, C., Dahl, A. C. & Retterstøl, N. (Red) (1980). *Gaustad Sykehus* 125 *År*. Oslo: Universitetsförlaget.

Barton, R. (1976). *Institutional neurosis*, 3rd ed. Bristol: John Wright & Son.

Brown, B. S. (1975). *De-institutionalization and Community Support Systems* (statement by the Director). NIMH (mimeographed).

Caffey, E. M., Galbrecht, C. R. & Klett, C. J. (1971). Brief hospitalization and aftercare in the treatment of schizophrenia. *Archives of General Psychiatry*, **24**, 81–6.

Caffey, E. M., Jones, R. D. & Diamons, L. S. (1968). Brief hospital treatment of schizophrenia: early results of a multiple hospital study. *Hospital and Community Psychiatry*, **19**, 282–7.

Davis, J. E. (1962). Family care of the mentally ill in Norway. *American Journal of Psychiatry*, **119**, 154–8.
Deutsch, A. (1949). *The Mentally Ill in America*. New York: Columbia University Press.
Fairweather, G. W. (ed.) (1964). *Social Psychology in Treating Mental Illness*. New York: J. Wiley & Sons Inc.
Foucault, M. (1965). *Madness and Civilization*. Garden City, New York: Doubleday.
Glick, I., Hargreawes, W. & Goldfield, M. (1974). Short versus long hospitalization. *Archives of General Psychiatry*, **30**, 363–9.
Goffman, E. (1961). *Asylums*. Garden City, New York: Doubleday.
Gottesfeld, H. (1977). *Alternatives to Psychiatric Hospitalization*. New York: Gardner Press Inc.
Gruenberg, E. M. (1966). Evaluating the effectiveness of mental health services. *Milbank Memorial Fund*, p. 44.
Gruenberg, E. (1967). The social breakdown syndrome: some origins. *American Journal of Psychiatry*, **123**, 1481–9.
Helgason, T. (1982). Alternatives to institutional psychiatric care in Iceland: changes in organization. Read at the *International Symposium on Alternatives to Institutional Psychiatric Care – Issues of Evaluation*, March 17, Umeå, Sweden.
Herz, M. I., Endicott, J. & Gibbon, M. (1979). Brief hospitalization: a two year follow-up. *American Journal of Psychiatry*, **134**, 502–7.
Honigfeld, G. & Gillis, R. (1967). The role of institutionalization in the natural history of schizophrenia. *Diseases of the Nervous System*, **28**, 660–3.
Jones, K. (1972). *A History of Mental Health Services*. London: Routledge & Kegan Paul.
Karno, M. & Schwarz, D. A. (1974). *Community Mental Health: Reflections and Explorations*. New York: Spectrum Publications.
Kernberg, O. (1981). Psychiatric hospital treatment in the United States. *Nordisk Psykiatrisk Tidsskrift*, **35**, 283–98.
Lee, D. T. (1963). Family care: selection and prediction. *American Journal of Psychiatry*, **120**, 561–6.
Morrissey, J. R. (1967). The case for family care of the mentally ill. *Community Mental Health Journal*, Monograph 2.
Paul, G. L. (1969). Chronic mental patient: current status – future directions. *Psychological Bulletin*, **71**, 81–94.
Perris, C. (1966). Community psychiatric service and aftercare of the patients returned to the community in the organization of a Swedish mental hospital. *International Journal of Social Psychiatry*, **12**, 293–8.
Perris, C., Kemali, D., Stancati, G. & Amati, A. (1984). Är den italienska reformlagen gällande psykiatrin mogen för motreform? *Nordisk Psykiatrisk Tidsskrift*, **38**, 364–77.
Regier, D. A. & Taube, C. A. (1981). The delivery of mental health services. In *American Handbook of Psychiatry*, 2nd edn, vol. 7, ed. S. Arieti & H. K. H. Brodie, pp. 714–33. New York: Basic Books.
Retterstøl, N. (1974). *Det Psykiatriske Sykehus i Omforming*. Oslo: Universitetsförlaget.
Segal, S. P. & Aviram, U. (1978). *The mentally ill in community-based sheltered care*. New York: J. Wiley & Sons Inc.
Socialstyrelsen anser (1980). *Riktlinjer för 80-talets Psykiatriska Vård*. No. 2, 1980.
SPRI (1982). *Utveckling av 80-talets allmänpsykiatri*. SPRI-rapport No. 75, 1982.
Test, M. A. & Stein, L. I. (1975). The clinical rationale for community treatment: a review of the literature. In *Alternatives to Mental Hospital Treatment*, ed. L. I. Stein & M. A. Test, pp. 3–22. New York: Plenum Press.
Wing, J. K. (1962). Institutionalism in mental hospitals. *British Journal of Social & Clinical Psychology*, **1**, 38–51.
Wing, J. K. & Hailey, A. M. (eds) (1972). *Evaluating a Community Psychiatric Service*. London: Oxford University Press.

The closing of mental hospitals in Italy and its impact on long-term treatment of functional psychoses

E. TORRE

Introduction

A new law enacted in May 1978, has significantly modified the Italian system of psychiatric patient care. The essential features of the new reform are: (*a*) since the date of the new act no 'first ever' has been admitted to a mental hospital as an in-patient (since July 1980, in our catchment area and in many other regions of the country, readmissions have also been prohibited); (*b*) all residential treatments, both compulsory and voluntary, have been undertaken in small psychiatric wards attached to general hospitals (the units have been established with an approximative ratio of 0.15 beds per 1000 population); (*c*) it has been suggested that the greater part of long- and short-term care should be assigned to out-patient departments, and local health authorities have been invited to implement the resources for non-residential services.

The new organization of the psychiatric care system was inserted into an ongoing process which started many years before, and has produced a decline of patients resident in the large mental hospitas; moreover, in some instances, sporadic efforts have been carried out towards a comprehensive community-oriented mental health service.

In this context, the closing of Italian hospitals means: (*a*) the construction of new large mental hospitals is prohibited; (*b*) although new admissions to mental hospitals are not allowed, some people (mostly long-stay in-patients suffering from functional psychoses) continue to live in the large traditional hospitals; (*c*) there are psychiatric wards attached to general hospitals which deliver short-term residential treatments.

As regards long-term care for patients suffering from functional psychoses, at present it might be assumed that the most relevant characteristics of the Italian care system are: (*a*) a marked reduction in bed numbers for residential treatment, especially for those patients needing more than a 2–3 months' stay; (*b*) a shortage of alternative settings (day hospitals, supervised hostels, group homes, etc.), unless old places with the same patients, now called 'guests', could be considered alternative facilities; (*c*) profound differences between regions and provinces, especially between the North and South, as to the phasing of the deinstitutionalization programme and the implementation of the new law.

Case-register studies

The background of this report was provided by evaluative studies carried out using a psychiatric case register. At the beginning, the studies concerned a health area near Pavia in Lombardia, a region of northern Italy (Torre, Marinoni & Allegri, 1982*a*; Torre *et al.*, 1982*b*; Marinoni *et al.*, 1983).

Subsequently, some colleagues (trained by the Mental Hygiene Unit of the University of Pavia) set up case-register procedures in three health areas of other regions of northern Italy, and comparisons of statistics were made (Ebbli & Bonizzoni, 1983; Torre *et al.*, 1983*a*, 1983*b*).

Information concerning the utilization of mental health services from a total population of about 300000 inhabitants (0.5% of the total Italian population) was available, on the basis of which tentative recommendations for local-service innovations could be made. Even though conclusions from these data are too parochial for generalizations to be made on the national level, ideas can be generated and hypotheses discussed.

Some sociodemographic characteristics of the health areas are summarized in Table 1. Sestri is a district in a large town (Genova) in Liguria; Lomest is a medium-sized town in Lombardia; Albenga in Liguria and Novi in Piemonte are areas comprising a small town (less than 20000 inhabitants) and many small rural villages. As would be expected, agricultural workers comprise about 20–5% of the population in Albenga and Novi, but are not significantly represented in the larger towns. In each area the percentage of economically active population is higher than the national mean, which is about 33%.

The mental hospital of each area lies outside its respective zone; the general hospital psychiatric unit is located within the area itself in Sestri and Novi, but about 65 km away from Lomest and Albenga. The out-patient service for Lomest has been operating since 1975, and since 1979–80 for the other areas.

Overall figures of the distribution of various types of care in the areas are provided in Table 2. The 1-year prevalance rates include four components: (*a*) in-patients on census day (December 31, of the previous

Table 1. *Socio-demographic characteristics of four areas in northern Italy (1971)*

	Lomest	Albenga	Novi	Sestri
Total population	80838	52548	77298	86187
Inhabitants per km²	486	174	105	4100
Males/females	0.93	0.96	0.94	0.94
Aged 0–14 (%)	20	18	17	19
Aged 65+ (%)	13	16	18	14
Economically active (aged 15+; %)	42	47	56	43
Occupation				
Agriculture (%)	2	24	18	1
Manufacturing (%)	67	26	50	55
Trade and services (%)	31	50	32	44

year); (*b*) patients who make contact with the hospital during the year following the census day; (*c*) out-patients actually attending the non-residential service before and after census day with no more than 3 months between attendances; (*d*) patients who make contact with the out-patient department during the year following the census day. The distribution of various types of contact is not homogeneous and Fig. 1 shows the different patterns graphically.

It seems that average estimates are more confusing than illuminating; moreover, it can be assumed that many factors are contributing to the trends in the various areas, such as a different impact of the deinstitutionalization programme, sociodemographic characteristics of the zones, the distance from residential settings, and the more or less community-oriented policy of the services. The relative weight of these factors upon different distributions of care might be a first issue for further research, both in general and specifically for patients suffering from functional psychoses needing long-term treatment. In this respect, collaborative projects among different countries might produce useful information for the more rational utilization of new resources, even though the actual allocation of money to health care services does not seem a first priority of many governments.

The majority of patients in hospital on census day will be long-stay patients (1 year or more in hospital) the number of elderly increasing with increasing rates of in-patients; schizophrenia is by far the most common diagnosis for both sexes. Fig. 2 shows the comparison of attrition numbers of long-stay in-patients from three areas. It seems realistic to assume that

Table 2. *One-year prevalence (1981) for various types of contact in four areas: rates per 100000 population aged 15+*

	Lomest	Albenga	Novi	Sestri
A: In-patient on 31 December of previous year	68	73	106	164
B: Not A, but admitted during the year	81	97	153	190
C: Not A and B, but out-patient on 31 December of previous year	214	50	206	170
D: Not A, B and C, but out-patient contact during the year	436	228	233	360
Total	799	448	692	884

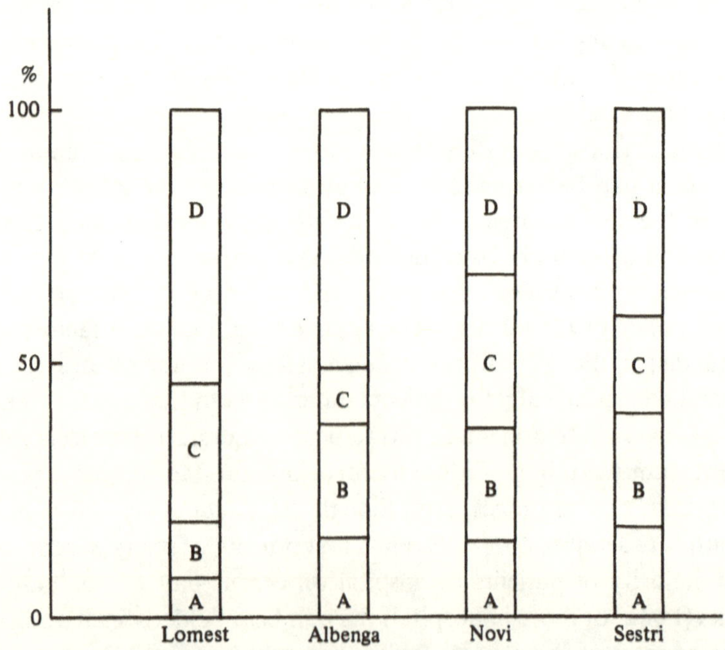

Fig. 1. Total patient population (1981) in four areas, by types of contact with in- and out-patient facilities (A, B, C, D as in Table 2).

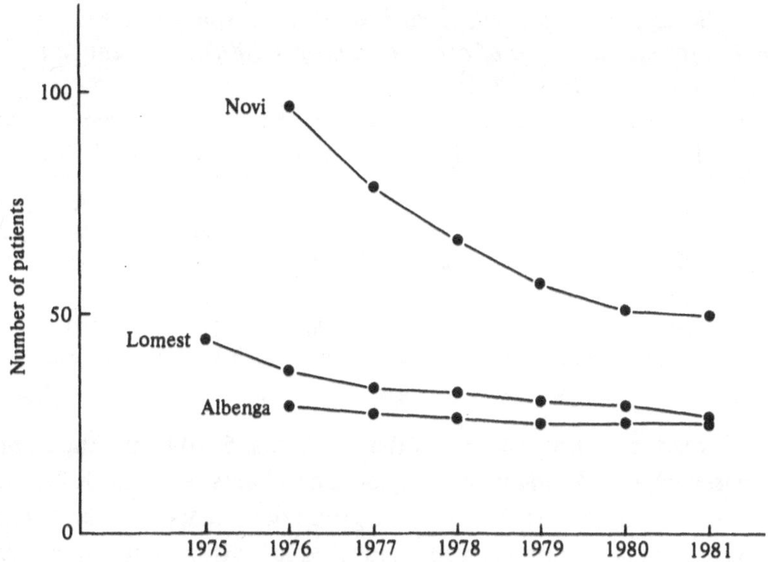

Fig. 2. Decline in number of old long-stay patients.

the old long-stay in-patients will remain a heavy load on the mental health care system for a long time; however, the new organization has stopped the build-up of new long-stay in-patients and their numbers cannot increase.

Hence, the question arises as to where and how patients needing long-term treatment will accumulate after the closing of hospitals. A preliminary answer may be based on three sets of data which refer to the build-up of high-user patients in the services. Obviously, the definition of these patients is arbitrary, and therefore operational statements have been tentatively investigated.

(1) The high-user group of out-patients are those who were in continuous contact with the out-patient department for 1 year or more with a maximum period of 3 months between attendances. Between 1976 and 1978, 762 patients were recorded on the Lomest case-register list; of these patients, 69 satisfied the established criteria. Almost all of them were patients previously discharged from the hospital; 2 out of 3 were classified as suffering from schizophrenia or affective psychoses. It seems that before the new reform, about 10% of the patients utilizing mental health services became people in prolonged contact with the conventional out-patient clinics. In the meantime, another type of accumulation was in progress in the hospital, that is, new long-stay patients (Hailey, 1974; Wing & Fryers, 1976; Howat, 1979; Talbot, 1979; (Babiker, 1980; Häfner & Klug, 1982).

(2) During 1977, 182 'new on the register' patients (2.8 per thousand)

Table 3. *Schizophrenic patients from Lomest. 1-year prevalence (1976–81) for various types of contact: rates per 100000 population aged 15+ (A, B, C, D as in Table 2)*

	1976	1977	1978	1979	1980	1981
A	40	37	43	40	42	40
B	54	56	34	48	48	38
C	60	62	42	25	59	64
D	33	36	68	73	59	51
Total	187	191	187	186	208	193

were recorded from Lomest, and of these patients, 55 (0.85 per thousand) were classified as suffering from functional psychoses. A 4-year follow-up study was carried out and the high-user group of patients were those who, at no more than 3-month intervals, made frequent visits to the out-patient clinics and occasionally were admitted to the hospital, usually to the small ward within the general hospital. Of the 55 psychotic patients, 50% were in continuous long-term care during the 4 years following their first contact with the services, but 30% disappeared after 1 or 2 contacts, even though clinical conditions were similar.

It seems that in the years after the new law, the majority of patients with a diagnosis of functional psychosis take one of two roads: a career as 'revolving door' patients (Bassuk, 1980) within the services and they do not seem to differ significantly from the new long-stay patients who accumulated before the act; or they break off contact with the services. Assuming that it is unrealistic to consider the latter (many of them, at least) as greatly improved after only one or two attendances, they probably become patients 'falling between the cracks' of a poorly integrated health care network. The problem is that it is difficult to forecast at the first assessment, who will take which road, and why; this might be another issue to be faced by a joint action of some research groups.

In 1976 the 1-year prevalence rate of schizophrenics from Lomest was 1.87 per thousand population aged 15 and over (Table 3), corresponding to 121 patients. Between 1977 and 1981, 57 new cases of schizophrenia were recorded on the register. In 1981 the rate was 1.93 and the number 125; of these patients, 81 were the same people recorded in 1976. In 1981, the patients not in care were: 40 from the 1976 group plus 13 from the 57 new cases accumulated between 1977 and 1981. These data seem to be a good replication of the previous survey. In effect, more than 50% of patients became chronic attenders of the services and about 30% dropped quickly out of care.

Further research

The purpose of this volume is to stimulate new research and to ask more precise questions on long-term treatment of functional psychoses. Usually, to raise new issues is a fascinating task, but to establish priorities is more difficult and to select between empirical projects involves even heavier responsibility. Therefore, I will suggest just three questions which are at present starting points for surveys in progress or might become aims of future collaborative studies.

There are indications that severe, psychotic patients after their first contact with services split into two groups, i.e. those who become patients in prolonged contact (Edwards & Carter, 1978; Sturt, Wikes & Creer, 1982) and those who disappear after a few attendances; but, to say *a priori* who will become a member of which category is hazardous. Is it possible at the first assessment to discriminate between the two? Are there reliable criteria of assessment and outcome? Is it possible to plan collaborative follow-up studies on this issue in order to minimize costs and permit small, financially limited research groups to face the problem?

There is a good deal of information about relationships between long-stay periods in the hospital and institutionalism, and there are some indications that high-user groups of patients show symptoms of high dependency on new residential or non-residential psychiatric settings. Is it possible to modify assessment methods for the old institutionalism into new procedures more fitting the characteristics of the new dependency?

The opening of non-residential psychiatric services and their closeness to the patient's home provide easier access to the various levels of care within local communities (Keane & Fahy, 1982). As a consequence of this, there are indications that some severe, chronic psychotic patients living at home outside the network of care and having social contacts exclusively with their relatives, now feel drawn to psychiatric services. From a certain point of view, they may be considered as people suffering from institutionalism but outside psychiatric institutional facilities. It would be useful to verify if these types of patients are few and accidental, or if they represent a consistent subgroup of chronic psychotics. In the latter case, it would be valuable to learn from the patients and their relatives what means they devised for coping with the effects of the psychosis without assistance from the psychiatrist.

There may be more relevant issues and more precise questions, of course;

perhaps the problems raised in this chapter are more representative of my own limits than of lacunae in the present state of knowledge.

Acknowledgements
The author is grateful to Professor A. Marinoni and Dr D. Ebbli, Dr G. Allegri, Dr P. Bonizzoni, and Dr C. Girardengo for their helpful comments and criticism.

References

Babiker, I. E. (1980). Social and clinical correlates of new long-stay. *Acta Psychiatrica Scandinavica*, **61**, 365–75.

Bassuk, E. L. (1980). The impact of deinstitutionalization on the general hospital psychiatric emergency ward. *Hospital and Community Psychiatry*, **31**, 622–7.

Ebbli, D. & Bonizzoni, P. (1983). Prime valutazioni dei servizi psichiatrici di due aree sanitarie della regione Liguria: l'Albenganese e Genova I. *Formazione Psichiatrica*. **4**, 129–41.

Edwards, C. & Carter, J. (1978). Day services and mentally ill. In *Community Care for Mentally Disabled*, ed. J. K. Wing & E. Olsen. Oxford: Oxford University Press.

Häfner, H. & Klug, J. (1982). The impact of an expanding community mental health service on patterns of bed usage: evaluation of a four-year period of implementation. *Psychological Medicine*, **12**, 177–90.

Hailey, A. M. (1974). The new chronic psychiatric population. *British Journal of Preventive Social Medicine*, **28**, 180–6.

Howat, J. (1979). Nottingham and the hospital plan: a follow-up study of long-stay inpatients. *British Journal of Psychiatry*, **135**, 42–51.

Keane, P. & Fahy, T. J. (1982). Who receives the aftercare? Utilization of services by discharged inpatients. *Psychological Medicine*, **12**, 891–902.

Marinoni, A., Torre, E., Allegri, G. & Comelli, M. (1983). Lomest psychiatric case register: the statistical context required for planning. *Acta Psychiatrica Scandinavica*, **67**, 109–17.

Sturt, E., Wikes, T. & Creer, C. (1982). A survey of long-term users of the community psychiatric services in Camberwell. In *Long-term Community Care: Experience in a London Borough*, ed. J. K. Wing. *Psychological Medicine*, Monograph Supplement 2.

Talbot, J. A. (1979). Care of the chronically mentally ill. Still a national disgrace. *American Journal of Psychiatry*, **136**, 688–9.

Torre, E., Ebbli, D., Marinoni, A., Allegri, G., Ciancaglini, P. & Castelnovi, C. (1983*a*), I registri dei casi psichiatrici di Lomest e dell'Albenganese: confronto di dati per la valutazione dei servizi. *Rivista Sperimentale de Freniatria*, **107**, 47–59.

Torre, E., Marinoni, A. & Allegri, G. (1982*a*). Lomest psychiatric case register: old and new long-stay patients. *Social Psychiatry*, **17**, 125–31.

Torre, E., Marinoni, A. & Allegri, G., Bosso, A., Ebbli, D. & Gorrini, M. (1982*b*). Trends in admissions before and after an act abolishing mental hospitals: a survey in three areas of northern Italy. *Comprehensive Psychiatry*, **23**, 227–32.

Torre, E., Marinoni, A., Girardengo, C., Scoglia, G., Oberti, I. & Demicheli, V. (1983*b*). Uno studio comparativo dell'utenza dei servizi psichiatrici di due aree sanitarie: i registri di Lomest e del Novese. *Formazione Psichiatrica*, **4**, 95–109.

Wing, J. K. & Fryers, T. (1976). *Psychiatric services in Camberwell and Salford.* Statistics from the Camberwell and Salford psychiatric registers. London: Institute of Psychiatry and Manchester: Department of Community Medicine, University of Manchester.

Future developments in Italy

R. MISITI

The psychiatric care reform law is still very unequally applied. Striking differences exist between geographic areas in the amount and type of services provided.

Trends in time

During the first year after this reform, about 10000 in-patients were discharged from mental hospitals. This represented a major acceleration of an already current tendency.

The decrease in psychiatric in-patients was greater in southern than in northern Italy and was rather small in areas where the deinstitutionalization process was already developed. This result was facilitated by the fact that in the mental hospitals there were many 'inmates' who were not psychiatric cases *sensu stricto*. However, episodes of neglect and abandonment were not rare; some people were discharged or sent to their areas of origin without the families being helped or before community services had been set up. How many such cases there were, we do not know. In the following years, discharges decreased to about 3000–4000 per year.

New services

The small units in the general hospital (Diagnosis and Treatment Services, DTS) were fairly rapidly organized; the norm, in most areas of northern and central Italy, being 15 beds per 100000 of the population. There have been long delays in the development of community services, especially of sheltered accommodation, group homes, social centres and sheltered work. No real relationship can be discerned between the discharge rate and the development of new services; on the contrary, the general impression given is the greater the number of discharges, the poorer the new services. Lack of rational planning is apparent.

Local variability

There are striking differences not only from region to region in Italy (the region, as an administrative unit, can legislate in health matters), but also among Local Health Units and within big cities. The main causes are political and cultural more than structural or financial. This large variability is likely to continue; 40% of the Italian provinces have not fully implemented even the 1904 law.

Patterns of care

It is possible to distinguish between three basic patterns of care.

Psychiatric hospitals plus Diagnosis and Treatment Services

New community services have not been developed. Only the emergency units (DTS) in general hospitals have been opened. There is practically no follow-up care for patients discharged from the psychiatric hospitals (PH). DTSs play a role of pure sedation, because of heavy pressure from unfiltered demand. Turnover rate is very high; psychotropic drugs are used almost exclusively. Staff are dissatisfied and frustrated.

New long-stay 'total' institutions sometimes reappear without a psychiatric label. They are variously called: nursing homes, old peoples homes, private treatment homes (*case di cura*). This pattern, still prevalent in the South, is now slowly changing toward the model described below.

Psychiatric hospitals plus Diagnosis and Treatment Services plus out-patient clinics

This model of care, while seemingly satisfying the main stipulations of the reform law, still betrays its true intent.

Some out-patient clinics are added to the DTSs. They are not usually integrated with the in-patient units and have different types of clients. They are open only a few hours each day, do not usually deal with 'crisis' situations and do not have workshops, meal services, day-hospitals, night accommodation, or training centres.

This model is prevalent in large cities. Most of the drawbacks described in the previous section still pertain (overcrowding of the DTS, neglect of in-patients, and so on). In some towns, like Rome and Naples, there has recently been an increase in 'compulsory treatment'. It has to be stressed that this happens in towns where, immediately after the institution of the reform law, 'compulsory admissions' had shown a 40% decrease.

Psychiatric hospitals plus Diagnosis and Treatment Services plus community centres

With this type of organization there is a comprehensive and integrated network of services based on the community centres. Patients may stay all day long in the centres; night accommodation for a few people is sometimes available. Sheltered flats, group homes, small residential communities have been developed. There are good links with general practitioners, the general hospital departments, the emergency services and the police. Much care is delivered in the patients' homes.

In the pattern described here, most contacts between patients and caregivers take place in out-patient clinics and are characterized by the use of traditional medical supports (psychopharmacological treatments, counselling, psychotherapy). Home visits are frequent (30% of all the contacts in Trieste) and 'social' interventions (trying both to find a place for patients to live, either an apartment or a boarding house, and obtaining a job or suitable training) are more common.

The future

Most services will probably move towards a model which is intermediate between the second and third patterns described above. This would be expected to overcome the most striking defects and gaps of previous systems; the spirit of the reform law will not be fully implemented in any case.

The goal of this intermediate model would be to ameliorate care in terms of quality and not only in terms of the amount of services, however well structured. According to this model, community centres will have support facilities (day-hospital, emergency beds, sheltered housing); domiciliary work will increase; referrals from general hospital departments and DTS will be rare. However, even when this model has been applied, psychiatric hospitals will not disappear either as a structure or as an 'idea' belonging to people's general mentality. Community work does not *per se* defeat institutional neglect or abandonment in the community, as is shown also by the US experience.

Quality of treatment and staff motivation become of paramount importance; new problems arise. In order to identify and overcome these difficulties a new pluriannual research project has been developed to establish methods and tools for health service evaluation. This will allow us to make even finer distinctions.

Conclusions

In the next few years there will be a rationalization of psychiatric care in Italy, which will be mainly positive but sometimes negative. The so-called antipsychiatric movement is likely to receive only minority support. Professional roles will tend to become better defined but also more rigid. However, the leading principle of the reform law will continue to motivate experiments, and will be a continuing source of criticism and stimulation.

A. Gramsci, an Italian politican and writer, used to say that in order to change for the better one needs both the pessimism of reason and the optimism of the will. It is easy to conclude with Stahler that

> For a majority of the most severely mentally disabled, rehabilitation, in the sense of achieving competitive employment, high social levels and a general return to the 'mainstream' of society [*sic*], is probably not, according to current knowledge, a realistic goal. Unfortunately, it is just these patients, whose needs are greatest, who typically receive the least attention in community-based programs.... We must accept the fact that, in focussing on a chronically disabled population, we are dealing with a group of marginal persons, a large percentage of whom are probably not able to become part of the mainstream of our society. Traditional concepts of prevention and rehabilitation have, at best, limited relevance for much of the target population of deinstitutionalization. Thus, it is important that we develop and utilize evaluation techniques that do not presuppose the elimination of mental illness and do not rely on standard concepts of progress to measure the outcome of program for those patients who can, at best, move only very slowly, perhaps almost imperceptibly. If we can 'only' improve the quality of life for the most seriously disabled by enhancing their comfort in acceptable out-of-hospital environments where they may proceed at their own pace, if we can accept the chronically mentally ill for what they are, and not for what we think they should be – we should perhaps be taking an undramatic, but important step forward in achieving the basic goal of humanizing care for chronic mental patients.

But this pessimistic realism may often conceal the lack of a desire to change and a lack of commitment in working towards as much autonomy and acceptance as possible for the individual patient.

Reference

Stahler, G. J. & Tash, W. R. (eds) (1982). Conceptual issues in the evaluation of the deinstitutionalization movements. In *Innovative Approaches to Mental Health Evaluation*. New York: Academic Press.

Optimal duration of long-term treatment in functional psychoses

R. SADOUN

Although the problem of optimal duration is always present in the mind of psychiatrists treating psychotic patients and is, in one or other of its various aspects, the subject of many publications, it is rarely considered as a whole.

Functional psychoses

It is generally accepted that functional psychoses consist of four main categories of psychotic disorders without any demonstrable organic aetiology: (*a*) affective psychoses, with manic-depressive psychosis as the main clinical entity; (*b*) schizophrenia, with its various clinical subcategories; (*c*) paranoid states of non-schizophrenic nature; and, (*d*) acute paranoid episodes frequently classified as acute schizophrenia. As conditions classified in the fourth category are by definition acute, they are not part of the question under discussion.

Long-term treatment

It is of course necessary to agree on the length of time implied by long-term. It can be suggested that it means at least 12–18 months.

Optimal duration

The notion of an optimal duration is itself closely linked to the objectives of psychiatric treatment. These objectives are the disappearance or alleviation of the symptoms and suffering of the patient, the correction of his pathological patterns of behaviour and the recovery of his best possible ability to function at the individual and social level.

The duration of treatment is considered optimal if these objectives are achieved in the shortest period of time. In practice, in the majority of cases, they can only partially be attained and the results are only relatively good.

Modern psychiatry has at its disposal a wide spectrum of therapeutic means ranging from specific antidepressant, antimanic and antischizophrenic drugs on the one hand, to a wide range of psychotherapeutic, institutional and community-care possibilities on the other, whose development has paralleled that of modern biological treatments.

As a rule, in modern psychiatry, the combined use of all available methods (either simultaneously or in succession) leads to better results than the best results obtained from any one of them alone. Despite this fairly well established fact, therapeutic creeds or preferences frequently lead to the misuse or abuse of one or other of these modern therapies.

Affective psychoses

The characteristic clinical feature of manic-depressive psychosis, the main clinical entity of this category of functional psychoses, is the occurrence at variable intervals of manic or depressive episodes in the bipolar type, or of depressive episodes alone in the unipolar type.

Depressive episodes are now treated by antidepressant drugs, manic episodes by neuroleptics and, more recently, by lithium carbonate. The need to administer these therapies over prolonged periods may be due to some biological resistance such as a failure to build up adequate blood levels. The way of handling these cases is well known. Although this problem is not exactly within the scope of this chapter, it must be stressed that criteria for interrupting antidepressant therapy and replacing it by other therapeutic methods, such as electroconvulsive therapy, are not yet sufficiently defined.

In affective psychoses, a long-term treatment is frequently given to prevent the recurrence of new episodes. This prevention is now achieved by lithium therapy or, in cases where lithium should be avoided, by preventive maintenance with antidepressants. Because of various side effects, the latter may be difficult to maintain over long periods.

In the case of lithium, which some clinicians consider to be a life-long treatment, the diagnostic criteria must be well established. Lithium therapy should be prescribed only if two relapses following a first episode have occurred in a period of time which is usually fixed at 18–24 months. The therapeutic-to-toxic margin of lithium is low. Constant clinical monitoring and blood tests must be conducted. Because of the risk of renal complications, the question of optimal duration must be extended to the need to establish the minimum effective daily dosage, in order to reduce the risk of kidney damage. More precise information needs to be established regarding this risk.

Sometimes, manic-depressive patients are reluctant to accept a life-long dependence on a drug which needs such continuous monitoring. This difficulty occurs especially in the case of those who benefit from the hypomanic phases in their personal, professional and creative life. There are obviously cases in which this reluctance should be accepted. In such patients, depressive episodes can be treated, when they occur, with appropriate antidepressants.

Usually, the treatment of major depressive conditions can be successfully achieved without hospitalization or with only a short stay in hospital. As we know, these short stays frequently exceed the critical period during which they are needed. Criteria for the optimal duration of these spells should be established more precisely.

Before leaving the subject of affective psychoses, we should bear in mind that numerous recent scientific studies have shown that some form of psychotherapy combined with the administration of drugs improves the final result.

Schizophrenia

With schizophrenia, the problem looks quite different because the course of the main clinical forms frequently consists of progressive episodes of variable duration. It is usually said that such episodes lead progressively to a state of mental impairment.

Modern drug therapy of schizophrenia is especially successful with florid forms which are accompanied by delusions and hallucinations (such as paranoid schizophrenia) and with schizophrenia of the schizoaffective type. On the other hand, cases in which the symptoms are ill-defined and mainly negative, such as withdrawal, apathy, loss of drive, are less responsive to drugs.

In considering the optimal duration, we should carefully take into account the pros and cons of maintaining the patient on antipsychotic drugs such as phenothiazines or butyrophenones. Extrapyramidal side effects usually prevented by antiparkinsonism agents, and especially tardive dyskinesia, could be better controlled if sensitive and simple assay measures of neuroleptic blood levels were at our disposal.

As we know, a history of relapse after the discontinuation of antipsychotics indicates the need for a longer-than-usual period of maintenance. Evidence of the ineffectiveness of antipsychotic drugs and evidence that their discontinuation does not lead to a relapse indicate the need for a gradual reduction of dosage leading to the termination of drug treatment. However, our clinical knowledge concerning these risks needs to be better established.

Specific methods such as the use of long-acting drugs, depot medication, drug holidays and the use of 'therapeutic windows' should also be discussed in terms of their influence on optimal duration.

Paranoid states

Most schools of psychiatry allocate to the category of paranoid states a variety of delusional conditions with a protracted course. In such cases, delusional beliefs are well systematized and the most common symptomatology consists of persecutory delusions based on ideas of reference, influence and jealousy. Here the personality remains intact or deteriorates minimally over a prolonged period of time. The disorders can be compatible with a satisfactory social adjustment for a long period of time and many of these individuals come to treatment only when, for some reason, their usual balance becomes disrupted. In these states, neuroleptics are more useful for their sedative effects than for their capacity to diminish the delusional ideas. In consequence, treatment is frequently of short duration. Psychotherapeutic and social interventions, supportive measures, when adequately performed, often prove more useful than is commonly acknowledged.

Because of their suspiciousness, these patients frequently have negative attitudes which make them reject any kind of psychiatric intervention before some serious behavioural disorder or criminal act leads to their legal commitment in a psychiatric institution.

Deinstitutionalization, community psychiatry and community support

Community psychiatry has been developed to avoid unnecessary long-term hospitalization, with its harmful effects on the possibilities of rehabilitation after a psychotic episode, especially in schizophrenics. This widely recommended policy has shown that an appreciable number of institutionalized patients were suffering more from this long-term hospitalization than from their mental disorders.

Community psychiatry recommends that the treatment of mental patients should be conducted as closely as possible to the patient's usual living conditions; that it should offer comprehensive services with a multidisciplinary approach, ensure a continuity of care by the same therapeutic team and work as much as possible to prevent the recurrence of disorders.

However, chronic mental patients who have had or are having long-term hospital care, can only be sent back to their community if a comprehensive range of ambulatory mental health services, including residential alternatives, are readily available. The frequent failure to provide these services leads to an appalling neglect of the chronically mentally ill.

Another important aspect of long-term treatment of functional psychoses consists of the negative consequences of drug side effects on the individual's ability to use the residual assets which could help him to play a positive role in the community. This point should not be neglected when the optimal duration of a drug treatment is assessed.

In many cases, no matter what long-lasting therapeutic efforts are made, patients are unable to adjust themselves to social life and to recover a sufficient degree of autonomy. The possibility of keeping them outside the hospital depends on the capacity of their family and friends to support them or on the ability of the psychiatric-care system to provide protective residential and living conditions other than those of the hospital. Too many programmes place upon the family or the community a burden which they quite understandably refuse to bear.

II: PATIENTS ASPECTS OF LONG-TERM TREATMENT

Needed areas of research in psychological treatments for functional psychoses

R. DALY

Interest in psychotherapy of the psychoses has waxed and waned. Freud (1953*a*, *b*, *c*) disagreed with Bleuler (1912) and Jung (1972) in their suggesting an organic aetiology of schizophrenia although he conceded that such a view did not exclude his own libido theory. Nevertheless Freud considered psychoses unsuitable for his new treatment.

> Psychoses, states of confusion and deeply-rooted (I might say toxic) depression are therefore not suitable for psycho-analysis; at least not for the method as it has been practised up to the present. I do not regard it as by any means impossible that by suitable changes in the method we may succeed in advancing beyond these hindrances – and so be able to initiate a psychotherapy of the psychoses. (Freud, 1953*c*)

Indeed during the years of high psychotherapeutic optimism, and preceding the widespread understanding and application of antipsychotic medication, considerable advances were made in intensive psychotherapy with schizophrenia, e.g. Fromm-Reichmann (1950) and Arieti (1955). Nevertheless during the past few decades psychotherapy has fallen into considerable decline as an important component in the long-term treatment of functional psychoses. Indeed the feeling has grown up that psychotherapy in these patients has negligible or even harmful effects. More often it is ignored as a treatment in this context (Wing & Wing, 1982). There has been a considerable renewal of interest in studying the effectiveness and efficiency of psychological treatments in psychiatry (Strupp & Bergin, 1969; Malan, 1973; Daly, 1981). In fact London & Klerman (1982) have made a plea for the urgent setting up of a national body in the United States, similar to the Food and Drugs Administration, to evaluate and regulate psychotherapies. They point out that psychotherapy costs in the United States are in excess of $1000000000, comparable with the expenditure on pharmacological treatments. In my own Health Board, the costs of paying personnel in mental hospitals exceeds the bill for medications by a large factor. Thus there surely is considerable justification for examining what these expensive personnel do and say during their encounters with schizophrenic patients, and what effect this may or may not have on the course of the illness of those suffering from chronic psychoses.

There are many classifications and definitions of psychotherapy. That of Dewald (1964) is widely quoted: 'a psychological process between two or more individuals, in which one (the therapist), by virtue of training and position, seeks systematically to apply psychological knowledge and interventions in an attempt to understand, influence and ultimately modify the psychic experience, mental function and behaviour of the other (the patient)'.

London & Klerman (1982) point to there being no satisfactory classifications of the psychotherapies, and indeed psychotherapy types are very numerous. Estimates suggest that there are 250 or more psychotherapies (Herink, 1980). Psychotherapy includes (*a*) psychoanalysis, which is obviously not feasible or suitable in this context; (*b*) purely verbal psychotherapies, such as psychodynamic psychotherapy (brief, long-term, individual, group, family, conjoint marital) and other miscellaneous therapies (psychodrama, cognitive therapy etc.); (*c*) behavioural therapies – desensitisation, flooding, modelling, social-skills training, biofeedback, relaxation training, self-management, self-monitoring, decision training etc.

The growth of consumerism, in general, and the Patients' Rights Movement, in relation to psychiatry, emphasizes the need to assay the benefits and risks of psychological treatments. Furthermore, the extensive change in the law in relation to involuntary treatment render grave responsibilities on those treating involuntary patients in relation to what is said and done to them during their period of confinement.

I have previously pointed out (Daly, 1981) in regard to the methodology in evaluating psychotherapy that it is important to conduct measurements in the following areas:

1. costs and benefits of psychotherapy;
2. knowledge and awareness of psychotherapy
   (*a*) amongst colleagues and
   (*b*) amongst the lay population;
3. the pain involved, which has to be treated in this population – this is after all, the task of psychotherapy;

4. the need for treatment;
5. who is capable of providing treatment (quality control) in relation to
   (*a*) professional training and
   (*b*) continuous assessment;
6. outcomes in psychotherapy.

Fortunately, paralleling the greatly increased number and variety of psychotherapies has been improvement in the technology of assessment.

Feinsilver & Gunderson (1972) pointed out that the requirements for research in the area of psychotherapy of the psychoses were (*a*) a well-defined population, (*b*) control groups in a comparative milieu, (*c*) a well-defined, relatively homogeneous and non-idiosyncratic therapeutic approach, (*d*) a carefully defined and selected group of therapists, and (*e*) measures of outcome which evaluate behaviour in a number of settings and take into account the patient's own subjective experience of himself, long-term treatment and follow-up. Strupp & Bergin (1969) have argued that only by considering multiple perspectives will it be possible to derive truly comprehensive evaluations of psychotherapy outcomes. Their tripartite model emphasized three perspectives:

1. that of the individual (patient);
2. the mental health profession;
3. society (family, neighbours, insurer or government).

Psychotherapists, early on, accepted that the treatment must be extensively remodelled for schizophrenic patients. Because the patient requires help in establishing an individual identity, the therapist must be supportive without making the patient dependent. The therapist must continually point out appropriate reality and avoid being drawn into responding in a maternal role. The frequent emergence of autistic material is met by reality-orientated comments, ignoring a large part of the fantasies, merely relating the affective components of the fantasies to the reality situation. Since any build-up of hostile transference feelings can disrupt the therapeutic relationship, the patient has to be confronted early on with the transference origins of such feelings.

Colby (1951) suggested that the psychotic ego attempts to heal itself by becoming neurotic. Therefore, the object of psychotherapy in schizophrenia is mainly supportive and adding to defences rather than uncovering. Emphasis is always placed on avoidance of magical or disturbing symbolism in the treatment of schizophrenic patients; lying on a couch is particularly to be avoided.

Most of the writings on psychotherapy with schizophrenia apply to non-hospitalized schizophrenic patients. Colby (1951) pointed to the danger of misdiagnosing schizophrenic patients and treating them in psychotherapy as neurotic patients.

Sullivan (1956) advised that the therapist should try to avoid collisions with the patient's self-esteem, anticipating an area explored by Leff *et al.* (1982). During psychodynamic psychotherapy with schizophrenics, silences are avoided, there is more activity and support by the therapist who, changing tactics, will break the silence with questions. And he will never (as in the treatment of neurotics) meet a question with a silence. He does not indulge in quizzing or probing and there is no prying into the thoughts of the psychotic patient. Similarly there is no uncovering of previous psychoses, and amnesias are left well alone, i.e. he continues to encourage repression. The traditional advice is that delusions should not be confirmed or denied. His task rather is to find areas of good ego function and to support these. The patient's fears of insanity or suicide or homicide must be frankly discussed and, in Colby's view, failure to do so is culpable negligence (we might bear in mind current litigation regarding the liability of the psychiatrist of President Reagan's would-be assassin).

Obviously practical advice has to be given, for example, avoidance of unnecessary plastic surgery, etc. Instinctual material, which comes out so readily with schizophrenics, has to be avoided and ignored; instead practical interpersonal difficulties are dealt with, as are problems with day-to-day living. The therapist has to build up the patient's trust in order that the patient accepts his views and explanations. It is considered wise to stop the psychotherapy if any persecutory delusions of the patient begin to involve the therapist.

Psychodynamic therapy of psychosis – its efficacy

Perhaps the best known and most methodologically rigorous study of psychotherapy and schizophrenia is that of Philip May (1968) at the Camarillo State Hospital. 228 subjects who met criteria for the diagnosis of schizophrenia were randomly assigned to five 20-bed wards where they received one of the following treatments:

1. psychotherapy,
2. psychotherapy plus drugs,
3. drugs,
4. electro-convulsive therapy (ECT),
5. milieu-therapy alone.

41 psychiatric residents and psychiatrists, with between 6 months and 6 years of experience, conducted the psychotherapy which was psychoan-

alytically oriented, ego supportive, and reality-defining with a minimum of depth interpretation. The patients were seen, on average, for 2 hours per week and were assessed at the end of 1 year. The total time in psychotherapy for each patient ranged from 7 to 87 hours, with a mean of 49 hours. Based on various test measures, psychotherapy plus drugs and drugs alone were shown to be (approximately equally) the most effective, while psychotherapy and milieu-therapy alone were (approximately equally) least effective. ECT was intermediate in effectiveness. Most reviewers have concluded since then that psychotherapy alone is a relatively ineffective treatment when compared to antipsychotic drugs. May's group compared the groups receiving drugs alone and that receiving psychotherapy plus drugs. There were very slight trends in favour of the latter group, but these were dismissed by the researchers as being insufficient to justify their provision economically. Thus they concluded that drugs alone was the most reasonable approach to meeting the needs of the majority of schizophrenics, and that psychotherapy was not indicated for the hospitalized schizophrenic patient, with or without drugs.

The therapist variable

Studies such as May's should make us think more of work such as that of Whitehorn & Betz (1954) who noted that some psychiatrists consistently did well with schizophrenic patients while others consistently did poorly. Their observations eventually led to the categorization of therapists into A and B types (Whitehorn & Betz, 1960). Therapists whose vocational interests resembled those of lawyers (Type A) seemed to do better with schizophrenic patients than those whose interest more closely resembled those of painters, mathematics and physical science teachers (Type B).

Individual versus group therapy

Luborski *et al.* (1971) reported that there were only two studies in the literature involving comparisons of individual with group psychotherapy for schizophrenic out-patients. They concluded that, overall, the comparisons showed that the gains from the two treatments were similar. O'Brien *et al.* (1972) conducted a controlled outcome study with 100 recently discharged schizophrenic patients. Basing their study on measures of social effectiveness and psychiatric ratings, they reported that group therapy produced significantly better outcome after 12 and 24 months of treatment than did individual psychotherapy. Rehospitalization rates did not differ significantly. Analysis of therapist variables failed to account for the differences in outcome.

The need exists for far more comparisons of group, individual and other treatments.

Behavioural treatment of chronic psychoses

There are of course, broadly speaking, two types of behaviour therapy: (*a*) that with a broad theoretical basis in learning and personality theory and (*b*) behaviour modification based on the operant conditioning of Skinner (1938), i.e. where behaviour is governed by feedback of its consequences. The task is (*a*) the analysis of behaviour, (*b*) the definition of the terminal behaviour sought and (*c*) the devising of schedules or programmes of learning where reinforcement is given for successively closer approximations to the target behaviour. Reinforcements must be effective and can consist of attention and praise or be negative or punitive. This calls for manipulation of the environment where novelty and good models are also important.

Behaviour therapy has been used extensively to reduce or control undesired behaviours in chronic psychotic patients.

Time out from positive reinforcement (TO) is a behaviour-modification technique in which positive reinforcers are withdrawn for a period of time following the undesirable behaviour. Bostow & Bailey (1969) found that brief periods of isolation, contingent on abusive talk by an institutionalized retarded adult, were effective in reducing the rate of that response. Haynes & Geddy (1973), using an own-control-replication paradigm, suggested from their results that TO (brief isolation in a small room for 10 minutes) could function as a punishing stimulus for the hallucinatory behaviours of psychotic adults.

Cognitive therapy

A new development within behaviour therapy is cognitive behaviour modification or cognitive behaviour therapy (Mahony, 1974). These methods assume that clinical disorders are the result of maladaptive or faulty thought patterns which can be identified and replaced with more adaptive cognitions. Cognitive behaviour modification is broadly divided into three types.

1. Rational-emotive therapy, where emotional disorders are seen as the consequence of specific irrational assumptions or self statements; treatment consists of verbal persuasion and logical argument directed towards altering the patient's irrational ideas.
2. Self-instructional training deriving from rational-emotive therapy and from the normal developmental sequence in which children

acquire internal speech and verbal-symbolic control over their behaviour. Maladaptive thoughts or self statements are identified; the therapist models appropriate behaviour while verbalizing problem-solving self-instructions; this is then applied by the patient.

3. Beck's (1976) cognitive therapy resembles the other methods but, in addition, Beck emphasizes the importance of behavioural approaches to altering the thought patterns. Procedures are designed to facilitate a more objective and detached view of anxiety-provoking events.

Clearly, there is a very wide scope for application of these new approaches to the long-term treatment of functional psychoses.

There is a tradition that psychiatric patients with systematized delusions are largely inaccessible to verbal modes of treatment. Slater & Roth (1969) suggest 'it is a waste of time to argue with a paranoid patient about his delusions'. But Milton, Patwa & Häfner (1978) provide an example of verbal intervention of an appropriate kind, substantially reducing overall psychiatric disturbance in a proportion of persistently deluded patients. They compared two techniques:

1. *Confrontation.* Here the technique was to be firm and consistent but polite in rejecting patients' beliefs, using phrases such as 'you are quite wrong'; 'I'm afraid there is no possible basis for your belief' and 'I would like to believe you but the whole idea is so ridiculous'. If the patient continued to express his beliefs the effort was made to persuade the patient that he must be wrong, otherwise he would not be in hospital. If the argument failed or the patient became too agitated, a move was made onto contemporary material topics.
2. *Belief modification.* Here an effort was made to deal with the least strongly held beliefs, and the therapist avoided disagreeing with the patient saying 'you may well be correct in your beliefs, but I would like to discuss them in more detail with you' etc. The therapist continued to outline possible alternative explanations for the belief, using approaches likely to prove acceptable to the patient.

They found that with regard to the strength of the delusion both treatments produced a slight fall after five sessions, with a further fall 6 weeks later in the belief-modification group. The improvement after 6 weeks was significantly greater in the belief-modification group than in the confrontation group. Both treatments also produced falls in scores on the Brief Psychiatric Rating Scale (BPRS). Non-significant ($p < 0.02$) changes were noted in social anxiety.

Meichenbaum & Cameron (1973) examined the efficacy of self-instructional training procedures in altering the attention, thinking and language behaviours of hospitalized schizophrenics. The first study was exploratory, designed to test the feasibility of training schizophrenics to self-instruct (SI) – initially aloud and, subsequently, to themselves – by means of cognitive modelling and cognitive rehearsal. It was found that the SI group improved with practice relative to assessment control groups, based on a digit-symbol-substitution task and on an auditory distraction digit-recall task.

The second study examined the therapeutic efficacy of extended individualized self-instructional training in changing a range of behaviours. The training emphasized practice in self-monitoring with a view to providing schizophrenics with cues for making appropriate self statements. The self-instructional group improved in relation to a practice control group on a variety of measures including the amount of 'healthy talk' produced in a structured interview, the level of proverb abstraction, level of perceptual integration of responses to an ink blot test and digit recall under distraction conditions. A major aspect of the treatment was training the schizophrenics not only to monitor their own behaviour and thinking, but to become more sensitive to the interpersonal facial and behavioural cues which others emitted when the patients manifested schizophrenic behaviours. The authors pointed out that the self statements used in their study were very generalized and future research ought to refine and construct self statement repertoires matched to the needs of different types of schizophrenic patients. They point out, for instance, that the cognitive strategies and tactical self-instructional manoeuvres (which a group of chronic non-paranoid process schizophrenics would need to rehearse) would be quite different from those required by a group of acute reactive paranoid schizophrenics.

Clearly, cognitive factors in behaviour modification are very important. The successes demonstrated for depressive disorders should encourage research with schizophrenic and other psychotic patients.

Argyle, Bryant & Trower (1974) have described social skills and have emphasized the importance of non-verbal communication. This is true, particularly for the chronic psychotic patients – modelling, role-playing and television playback have all been used extensively in this regard. The skills being sought in the structural-learning therapy for schizophrenics have been: beginning, participating in, and ending a conversation; making a complaint; asking for help; rehearsing stressful encounters; coping with aggression; planning and self-control. The treatment is often carried out in groups or individually, closed circuit television tapes are played as models; training, practice and rehearsal are carried out and therapists give corrective feedback and reinforcement via praise. Lastly, the behaviour must be transferred to the home situation through assigned homework. Ultimately self-management and self-control techniques are required by the patient. A problem has been of course that a high degree of cooperation is required of the patients, and in schizophrenia the cognitive deficits are extensive. Ayllon & Michael (1959) noticed undesirable effects of psychiatric nursing. The therapist in this case got the nurses to transfer their attention to desirable behaviours. Isaacs, Thomas & Goldiamond (1960) showed that it was possible, by using operant methods, to reinstitute speech in a mute patient who had been withdrawn for many years.

Token economies

From the simple idea of incentives and deterrents evolved the token-economy (TE) programmes, pioneered by Aylon & Azrin (1968). A large number of researchers have been generating increasingly complex programmes. Tokens were given which could then be used to purchase goods. Exponents of these methods sought 'purism' and counselled against complicating the TE environment by developing therapist–patient relationships.

There is increasing agreement that such a narrow approach is detrimental since cognitive processes play an important role in the acquisition and retention of new patterns of behaviour. There seems a need therefore to evolve more broadly based theoretical approaches in which TEs play a part, along with individual and group psychotherapy, as well as cognitive and behavioural approaches.

Personal construct theory

Bannister *et al.* (1975) considered that an individual's view of the world, and interpersonal relationships in particular, is influenced by his placing expectations along bipolar dimensions. These dimensions are a result of the individual's learning experience and are peculiar to him. The dimensions may be, for example, 'good or bad', 'honest or dishonest'. A person's construct system may be explored by means of Bannister's Repertory Grid Test. The Repertory Grid has also been used by Bannister to provide an operational definition of the thought disorder of schizophrenia. It attempts to measure the closeness of relationships between an individual's constructs and the consistency with which these constructs or expectations are maintained. Thought disorder is characterized by weak or inconsistent relationships between constructs. A normal person, for example, will have good relationships between constructs such as honest and good and dishonest and bad. Thought-disordered schizophrenics, on the other hand, show poor correlations. Bannister suggests that during the development of the schizophrenic patient, repeatedly invalidated constructs lead to vague and imprecise constructs, a phenomenon similar to Bateson *et al.* (1956) Double Bind. A great advantage of Bannister's theory is that it can be tested experimentally. Unfortunately the treatment he designed on the basis of this theory and testing does not seem to have been very effective in his initial trial. The treatment consists in long-term serial validation of such weak constructs to enable the patient to 'tighten' his perception of reality. In this research, the construct system of the long-stay patients was closely examined for islands of meaning within the general loose structures. This is followed by fortnightly sessions for 2 years aimed at validating and tightening these areas. It was also designed to extend relationships with neighbouring areas and to stabilize the network of constructs. Bannister himself felt that a greater degree of environmental control was required.

While personal constructs seem not to have generated useful psychological treatments they should nevertheless form part of the assessment resources of researchers studying psychological treatments.

Psychotherapy as an alternative to maintenance medication

Increasing dissatisfaction has arisen with the chronic use of neuroleptic medication. Despite their dramatic effectiveness, serious side effects occur, particularly tardive dyskinesia. Indeed, there is evidence that some patients receiving phenothiazine medication have impairment of vocalisation preceding the development of akinetic mutism (Behrman, 1972). Thus, for a very small number of patients ability to participate in psychological treatments may be impaired by pharmacological treatments. Research in this area should be carried out to identify and cope with this problem. Bleuler (1978) and others contend that the need for indefinite maintenance on neuroleptics was much overrated. Hogarty & Goldberg (1973) suggested that, for the majority of patients, the major function of antipsychotic drugs was to help prevent relapse. Obviously many patients show immediate deterioration on withdrawal from medication but intermittent medication is suitable for the many stable schizophrenic out-patients (Herz, Szymanski & Simon, 1982).

For such patients withdrawn from antipsychotic medication, considerable research is required into the effectiveness of various psychological treatments in preventing relapse.

Using new technology in communications.

A problem in dealing with chronic psychotic patients has been in relation to difficulties of communicating with them, and the related problem of treatment adherence. High drop-out rates are described in nearly all out-patient clinics, particularly for psychotic patients. Nevertheless very few reports describe utilization of modern communications technology in helping to overcome this problem. Turner & Vernon (1976) described substantial success in increasing the percentage of patients who kept their initial appointments by telephone reminders. They suggested financial advantages from assigned staff to carry this out. On the other hand Burgoyne, Acosta & Yamamoto (1983) concluded from their study that initial attendance at out-patient clinics appears more related to the socioeconomic level of the patients, i.e. their having a telephone rather than being telephoned. There may be non-causal relationships between telephoning and attendance at clinics.

Research should, however, be carried out, using telephonic or other communications technology, as a means of supportive psychotherapy or as a reinforcer of desirable behaviours. It has already been pointed out that psychotherapists dealing with schizophrenic patients need to be more widely available and less restrictive in their approaches. Telephones have been widely used in suicide-prevention services, and it would seem appropriate to test further the feasibility of such systems for chronic psychotic patients.

Psychophysiology and Treatment

Tarrier *et al.* (1979) tested schizophrenic patients on psychophysiological measures within their homes and in the laboratory. They found that sweat-gland activity and heart-rate changes occurring when patients encountered novel situations (life events), together with the home atmosphere generated by a critical or overinvolved relative, confirmed objectively the importance of previous social measurements of these factors in determining relapse. They found that responses to psychopharmacological treatments were also modified by these social factors.

Interestingly, environmentally and socially induced changes found in the home were not detectable in their laboratory. The same group (Sturgeon *et al.*, 1981) measured spontaneous fluctuations in skin conductance in acutely ill schizophrenic patients. These measures were carried out in a videotape studio. Recordings were made, initially with the patient talking to an interviewer, then during a videotaped interview conducted with the patient's key relative. The expressed motion of the patient's key relative had been measured previously. Far greater levels of spontaneous fluctuations were found with relatives present, and most dramatic of all was the high level of fluctuations found when relatives with high expressed emotion were present.

Obviously, further work in this area combining psychological factors with physiological measures needs to be carried out. The case has been made for managing the physiological responses of such patients. A particularly promising area lies in training them to cope with their physiological responses, via biofeedback, relaxation training and other such physiologically directed approaches. In addition, while separation from high expressed emotion relatives has been the key intervention, this is not always possible. Further work has therefore been carried out into the training of such relatives. It would also seem appropriate to train the patients to avoid stressful experiences via self-monitoring, self-management and self-control.

Compliance with research protocol

While much attention has been given to compliance with treatment in drug trials (via measuring blood levels of drugs) it has been assumed that in psychotherapy trials it is known who is and is not getting a particular 'dose' of treatment. However, Donovan (1977) in his study of psychological interventions in smoking and pregnancy found an 18% discrepancy between self-reporting of smoking during pregnancy and post-partum. He found that the group reported to get counselling via an elaborate scheme, turned out to get treatment in only 31% of cases. This proportion was not statistically different from controls who reported advice in the same proportion which they had received adventitiously. The problem, therefore, is of knowing who does and does not get psychological treatments. Many studies such as that of May (1968) have been criticized for the unquantifiable 'dose' of psychotherapy being applied in each case.

Weissman, Rounsaville & Chevron (1982) addressed themselves to this problem. They described the difficulties involved in training experienced psychotherapists to participate in outcome studies. They found the areas of conflict to be in relation to research goals, clinical goals and therapists' expectations. Restrictions were also imposed by the research protocol, the therapists' feelings about being evaluated and the restrictions of a defined psychotherapy. They suggested that a training programme that addresses itself to these problems, together with an appropriate administrative structure, could reduce such conflicts.

Quality of life

The recognition that chronic psychiatric patients suffer severe hardships in many life areas (such as housing, family environment, social networks, finance, safety and coping skills) has led Lehman (1983) to explore the concept of quality of life (QOL). He uses both subjective assessments and objective measures (such as income level) combined with ratings by others, to arrive at a measure of global wellbeing of chronic psychiatric patients. In his survey he found the following to be predictors of perceived global wellbeing:

1. whether or not the patient was victimized in a crime;
2. availability of medical care;
3. frequency of intimate social relationships during the previous year;
4. health satisfaction;
5. satisfaction with leisure time;
6. satisfaction with social relations;
7. satisfaction with finances.

From these results he suggested that further attention should be given to programmes designed (*a*) to improve patient safety in and around boarding homes and hostels: (*b*) to ensure that their utilization of health services is appropriate and to make available alternative services that meet the non-medical quality of life needs; (*c*) to enhance their social skills and opportunities for establishing more satisfying relationships, especially within the board and care homes; (*d*) to identify the types of daily activities, whether leisure- or work-related, that they find most satisfying; and (*e*) to improve their financial resources, e.g. through more realistic work opportunities or more generous entitlement programmes. Quality of life could be used more widely as a measure of clinical outcome and as a measure in cost-effectiveness studies.

Psychotherapy as prophylaxis in children

At the World Health Organization (WHO) Working Group entitled 'Primary prevention of schizophrenia in high risk groups' (WHO, 1977), Eisenberg was not enthusiastic about psychotherapy as prophylaxis for psychoses 'since present evidence indicated its low efficacy compared to anti-psychotic drugs'. In addition, he felt that there would be ethical problems in intervening with apparently normal children, particularly as psychotherapy was potentially 'toxic' (Eisenberg, 1975). Despite his reservations he still considered that when pathological symptoms appeared in children who were being followed such children merited treatment by the best available method.

He referred also to competence training (Anthony & Koupernick, 1974; Gamezy, 1974), describing programmes intended to enhance childrens' coping abilities. Again, Eisenberg was somewhat dubious about the specific preventive aspects of such interventions, but he felt that there was virtue in providing growth-promoting experiences for any child, particularly those who are in the deprived category. Finally, one must say that the long-term results of the Cambridge–Somerville Project cast serious doubts on the advisability of such interventions.

Psychotherapy and the defect state

Various writers since Kraepelin (1919) have reported impairment of intellectual functioning. Lilliston (1973) described three groups of schizophrenic patients, selected because of their poor performance on cerebral-damage tests. The group with the highest scores for brain damage were found to be at the process end of the process reactive dimension, had high scores on perceptual abnormality, showed less insight and poorer affect. They had in addition disorientation for time and space. Crowe & Mitchell (1975) found that a substantial number of chronic schizophrenic patients underestimated their own age and thought they had been in hospital for much briefer periods of time than they really had. It was felt that for such patients 'time stood still'.

More recently computerized axial tomography has demonstrated increased ventricular size, casting a somewhat surprising new light on the organic aspect of schizophrenia. It is possible that new individual and group psychotherapeutic approaches will follow these developments.

Leff *et al.* (1973) have pointed out that schizophrenic patients living in the community and not taking drugs seemed to relapse as a result of a disturbance of everyday social interactions. They have extensively explored this area of the influence of family life on the course of schizophrenia. Vaughn & Leff (1976) found that the index of emotion expressed by a key relative about the patient at the time of the admission proved to be the best single predicator of symptomatic relapse in the months after discharge from hospital. They also found important additive effects between various social influences and pharmacological treatments which made it possible to predict relapse patterns in schizophrenia with considerable precision. The patterns of these relationships with relapse are different for the two clinical groups.

In a further study (Leff *et al.*, 1982) the patients were all selected for being in close contact with high expressed emotion relatives. All patients were maintained on neuroleptic drugs. One half received the package of social interventions while the other half, on routine out-patient care, were assigned as controls. The package consisted of a programme of education about schizophrenia, a group for the relatives and family sessions for relatives and patients. The relapse rate in the control group was 50% compared with 9% in the experimental group. The stated aims of the therapeutic interventions were achieved in 73% of the experimental families, i.e. in these families no patient relapsed. The results provided clear evidence for a causal role of relatives' expressed emotion.

It would seem that expressed emotion may be used in studies of other functional psychoses, and possibly in other aspects of psychological treatment for schizophrenia, e.g. with measures applied to treatment staff.

Miscellaneous therapies

Another aspect of the Patients' Rights Movement and freedom of information legislation in the United States (a trend beginning in Europe) has been that patients may have access to their records. Roth, Wolford & Meisel (1980) have explored the effect of this on patients, and conclude that, far from harm being caused, it has generally been positive. They felt that one schizophrenic patient was harmed by not having access to her record. Nonetheless, records perhaps should be written with this in mind, and it is essential that staff are at hand to go through the record with the patient. An opportunity is available here for further research. In the past hypnosis and other uncovering treatments have not been thought to be appropriate for schizophrenic and functionally psychotic patients. However, Bliss, Larson & Nakashima (1983) studied 45 patients with auditory hallucinations, most of whom had been diagnosed as having schizophrenic or affective illness. Ten of their patients were incidentally treated with hypnotherapy, and multiple personalities were found in the ten cases. They suggest that although it is generally assumed that schizophrenics are poor hypnotic subjects the survey of the literature did not support such a generalization.

Conclusion

In summary, one might say that the task of researchers in psychological treatments for schizophrenia will be to devise new ways of tailoring treatments to suit individual needs. A start has been made by McGlashan (1982) using DSM III diagnoses to assign schizophrenic patients for varying types of psychodynamic therapy.

One of the most widely quoted reviews of evaluation of treatment in schizophrenia is that of May & Simpson (1980) who felt that techniques aimed at deep psychological understanding and insight were not helpful and that, for the majority of patients 'drug treatment speeds up the process of recovery, leads to a higher level of functioning, and reduces the risk of relapse. Nevertheless, drugs alone are not sufficient. Optimal treatment requires a mixture of pharmaco-therapy and social and psychological intervention'.

One might add that new measures (including cost effectiveness and novel psychometric techniques) and new psychological treatments have produced a widening field, demanding extensive research.

References

Anthony, E. J. & Koupernick, C. (1974). *The Child and his Family: Children at Psychiatric Risk*, pp. 77–97. New York: Wiley & Sons.

Argyle, M., Bryant, B. & Trower, P. (1974). Social skills training and psychotherapy: a comparative study. *Psychological Medicine*, **4**, 435–43.

Arleti, S. (1955). *Interpretation of Schizophrenia.* New York: Brunner.

Ayllon, T. & Azrin, N. H. (1968). *The Token Economy: a Motivational System for Therapy and Rehabilitation.* New York: Appleton-Century-Crofts.

Ayllon, T. & Michael, J. (1959). The psychiatric nurse as a behavioural engineer. *Journal of the Experimental Analysis of Behavior*, **2**, 323–34.

Bannister, D., Adams-Webber, J. R., Penn, W. I. & Radley, A. (1975). Reversing the process of thought disorder: a serial validation experiment. *British Journal of Social and Clinical Psychology*, **14**, 169–80.

Bateson, G., Jackson, D., Haley, J. & Weakland, J. (1956). Towards a theory of schizophrenia. *Behavioral Science*, **1**, 251–64.

Beck, A. T. (1976). *Cognitive Therapy and the Emotional Disorders.* New York: International University Press.

Behrman, S. (1972). Mutism induced by phenothiazines. *British Journal of Psychiatry*, **121**, 599–604.

Bleuler, E. (1912). The theory of schizophrenic negativism. *Nervous and Mental Disease*, Monograph, No. 11. New York: Nervous and Mental Disease Publishing Company.

Bleuler, M. (1978). *The Schizophrenic Disorders: Long-term Patient and Family Studies.* New Haven: Yale University Press.

Bliss, E. L., Larson, E. M. & Nakashima, S. R. (1983). Auditory hallucinations and schizophrenia. *Journal of Nervous and Mental Disease*, **171**, 30–3.

Bostow, D. E. & Bailey, J. B. (1969). Modification of severe disruptive and agrressive behaviour using brief time-out and reinforcement procedures. *Journal of Applied Behavior Analysis*, **12**, 31–8.

Burgoyne, R. W., Acosta, F. X. & Yamamoto, J. (1983). Telephone prompting to increase attendance at a psychiatric out-patient clinic. *American Journal of Psychiatry*, **140**, 345–7.

Colby, M. K. (1951). *A Primer for Psychotherapists.* New York: Wiley & Sons.

Crowe, T. J. & Mitchell, W. S. (1975). Subjective age in chronic schizophrenia: evidence for a sub-group of patients with defective learning capacity? *British Journal of Psychiatry*, **126**, 360–3.

Daly, R. J. (1981). Special problems in evaluation of psychotherapy. In *Methodology and Evaluation of Psychiatric Treatment*, EMRC Workshop, ed. T. Helgason, 123–36. Cambridge University Press.

Dewald, P. (1964). *Psychotherapy: a Dynamic Approach.* New York: Basic Books.

Donovan, J. W. (1977). Randomised controlled trial of anti-smoking advice in pregnancy. *British Journal of Preventive and Social Medicine*, **31**, 6–12.

Eisenberg, L. (1975). The ethics of intervention: acting amidst ambiguity. *Journal of Child Psychology and Psychiatry and Allied Disciplines*, **16**, 93–104.

Feinsilver, D. B. & Gunderson, J. G. (1972). Psychotherapy for schizophrenics – is it indicated? *Schizophrenia Bulletin*, **6**, 11–23.

Freud, S. (1953*a*). The loss of reality in neurosis and psychosis. *Collected Papers*, **11**, 277–82. London: The Hogarth Press.

Freud, S. (1953*b*). Neurosis and psychosis. *Collected Papers*, **11**, 250–4. London: The Hogarth Press.

Freud, S. (1953*c*). *Collected Papers*, **1**, p. 258, 312. London: The Hogarth Press.

Fromm-Reichmann, F. (1950). *Principles of Intensive Psychotherapy*. Chicago: University of Chicago Press.

Garmezy, N. (1974). The study of competence in children at risk for severe psychopathology. In *Child in His Family. Children at risk*, vol. 3, ed. E. J. Anthony & C. Koupernick, pp. 77–97, New York: Wiley & Sons.

Haynes, S. N. & Geddy, P. (1973). Suppression of psychotic hallucinations through time-out. *Behaviour Therapy*, **4**, 123–7.

Herink, R. (1980). *The Psychotherapy Handbook*. New York: New American Library.

Herz, M. I., Szymanski, H. M. & Simon, J. C. (1982). Intermittent medication for stable schizophrenic out-patients: an alternative to maintenance medication. *American Journal of Psychiatry*, **139**, 918–22.

Hogarty, G. E. & Goldberg, S. C. (1973). Drugs and socio-therapy in the post hospital maintenance of schizophrenic patients: 1-year relapse rates. *Archives of General Psychiatry*, **28**, 54.

Isaacs, W., Thomas, J. & Goldiamond, I. (1960). *Journal of Speech and Hearing Disorders*, **25**, 8–12.

Jung, C. G. (1972). *Collected Works*, vol. 3, pp. 233–49. Princeton: Princeton University Press.

Kraepelin, E. (1919). *Dementia Praecox* (translated by R. M. Barcley, facsimile edition). New York: R. E. Krieger, 1971.

Leff, J. P., Hirsch, S. R., Gaind, R., Rohde, P. D. & Stevens, B. C. (1973). Life events and maintenance therapy in schizophrenic relapse. *British Journal of Psychiatry*, **123**, 659–60.

Leff, J. P., Kuipers, L., Berkowitz, R., Eberlein-Vries, R. & Sturgeon, D. (1982). A controlled trial of social intervention in the families of schizophrenic patients. *British Journal of Psychiatry*, **141**, 121–34.

Lehman, A. F. (1983). The well-being of chronic mental patients. *Archives of General Psychiatry*, **40**, 369–73.

Lilliston, L. (1973). Schizophrenic symptomatology as a function of probability of cerebral damage. *Journal of Abnormal Psychology*, **82**, 377–81.

London, P. & Klerman, G. L. (1982). Evaluating psychotherapy. *American Journal of Psychiatry*, **139**, 709–17.

Luborsky, L., Chandler, M., Auerbach, A. N., Cohen, J. & Bachrach, H. M. (1971). Factors influencing the outcome of psychotherapy: a review of quantitative research. *Psychological Bulletin*, **75**, 145–85.

McGlashan, T. H. (1982). DSM-III schizophrenia and individual psychotherapy. *Journal of Nervous and Mental Disease*, **170**, 752–7.

Mahony, M. J. (1974). *Cognition and Behaviour Modification*. Cambridge, Mass.: Ballinger.

Malan, D. H. (1973). The outcome problem in psychotherapy research: a historical review. *Archives of General Psychiatry*, **29**, 719–29.

May, P. R. A. (1968). *Treatment of Schizophrenia: a Comparative Study of Five Treatment Methods*. New York: Science House.

May, P. R. A. & Simpson, G. M. (1980). Schizophrenia: Evolution of treatment methods. In *Comprehensive Textbook of Psychiatry*, vol. 3, 3rd edn, ed. H. I. Kaplan, A. M. Freedman & B. J. Sadock, pp. 1240–75. Baltimore: Williams & Wilkins.

Meichenbaum, D. & Cameron, R. (1973). Training schizophrenics to talk to themselves: a means of developing attention controls. *Behavior Therapy*, **4**, 515–34.

Milton, F., Patwa, V. K. & Häfner, R. J. (1978). Confrontation *vs* belief modification in persistently deluded patients. *British Journal of Medical Psychology*, **51**, 127–30.
O'Brien, C. P., Kyle, B., Ben, A., Pierce, J. F. (1972). Group *vs* individual psychotherapy with schizophrenics. *Archives of General Psychiatry*, **27**, 474–8.
Roth, L. H., Wolford, J. & Meisel, A. (1980). Patient access to records: tonic or toxin? *American Journal of Psychiatry*, **137**, 592–6.
Skinner, B. F. (1938). *The Behaviour of Organisms*. New York: Appleton-Century-Crofts.
Slater, E. & Roth, M. (1969). *Clinical Psychiatry*, p. 326. London: Baillière, Tindal & Cassell.
Strupp, H. H. & Bergin, A. (1969). Some empirical and conceptual bases for co-ordinated research in psychotherapy. *International Journal of Psychiatry*, **1**, 18–90.
Sturgeon, D., Kuipers, L., Berkowitz, R., Turpin, G. & Leff, J. (1981). Psychophysiological responses of schizophrenic patients to high and low expressed emotion relatives. *British Journal of Psychiatry*, **138**, 40–5.
Sullivan, H. S. (1956). *Clinical studies in Psychiatry*. New York: Norton.
Tarrier, N., Vaughn, C., Lader, M. H. & Leff, J. P. (1979). Bodily reactions to people and events in schizophrenics. *Archives of General Psychiatry*, **36**, 311–15.
Turner, A. J. & Vernon, J. C. (1976). Prompts to increase attendance in a community mental health centre. *Journal of Applied Behavior Analysis*, **9**, 141–5.
Vaughn, C. E. & Leff, J. P. (1976). The influence of family and social factors on the course of psychiatric illness: a comparison of schizophrenic and depressed neurotic patients. *British Journal of Psychiatry*, **129**, 125–57.
Weissman, M., Rounsaville, B. J. & Chevron, E. (1982). Training psychotherapists to participate in psychotherapy outcome studies. *American Journal of Psychiatry*, **139**, 1442–6.
Whitehorn, J. C. & Betz, B. J. (1954). A study of psychotherapeutic relationships between physicians and schizophrenic patients. *American Journal of Psychiatry*, **111**, 321–31.
Whitehorn, J. C. & Betz, B. J. (1960). Further studies of the doctor as a crucial variable in the outcome of treatment with schizophrenic patients. *American Journal of Psychiatry*, **117**, 214–23.
Wing, J. K. & Wing, L. (eds) (1982). Psychoses of uncertain aetiology. In *Handbook of Psychiatry*, vol. 3. Cambridge University Press.
World Health Organization (1977). Primary prevention of schizophrenia in high-risk groups. *Report on a Working Group*. Copenhagen: WHO ICP/MMH 026111.

Family therapy as part of the treatment of schizophrenia

Y. O. ALANEN

Need for comprehensive research approach to the treatment of schizophrenia

Schizophrenia treatment and research is hampered by a lack of integration of different conceptions as to the nature of the illness. Researchers have specialized in different fields, and even clinicians too often are restricted to a relatively narrow therapeutic orientation, with little knowledge of other approaches. We should, in my view, recognize the multidimensional nature of our task and aim at the further development of the treatment of schizophrenia; our approach should be integrated, but at the same time differentiated according to the individual case. I therefore consider it necessary to approach my own subject, research on family therapy, from a comprehensive viewpoint. The most important concepts of schizophrenia, and the treatment modes connected with them, are shown simplified in Fig. 1.

There is no need to consider in greater detail here the aetiological theories underlying these orientations. Instead I want to stress that each of these therapeutic approaches can be justified on the basis of research data; it has its own importance as a therapy, and its own limitations as well. Schizophrenic patients form a heterogeneous group in which therapeutic needs are individually weighted in different ways. This must be taken into account in planning the treatment in order to attain the best possible results (Alanen *et al.*, 1982*a*).

In research work too, more attention should be paid to a multi-dimensional approach. One weakness which can be seen in many treatment studies is a certain methodological rigidity in the theoretical framework itself. A group of schizophrenics is selected on random grounds, to receive a specific form of treatment; this is administered in a rigidly schematic manner while other similar groups, selected as controls, receive different

(1) *Biomedical model*
'the illness is comprehended as an organic brain process'
– psychopharmacological treatment
– other 'organic' treatments

(2) *Individual psychological model*
'the illness is based on a deep-rooted disorder of the personality development'
– individual psychotherapy

(3) *Transactional (systemic) model*
'the illness is part of a disordered interactional network'
– family therapy
– group- and community-based treatment systems

---

(4) *Larger social–psychiatric context*
'the patient must have support as a member of community'
– rehabilitation
– environment-centred mental health activities

The treatment should be developed in a global way according to case-specific needs

Fig. 1. Illness models of schizophrenia.

treatment or none at all. Such a research design does not lead to an adequate view of the possibilities of an individually planned psychotherapeutic treatment approach to schizophrenia (Alanen *et al.*, 1980). It may be more meaningful to study what case-specific clinical, family-dynamic and social-background variables should be taken as indications for a certain type of treatment, or for a treatment-mode combination weighted in a certain way. The indications of family-centred treatment modes should also be considered from such a comprehensive point of view, not as a treatment carried out separated from a more global treatment plan.

Why family therapy? Some developmental trends

Family-oriented treatment is needed in schizophrenia for many reasons. A psychotic breakdown on the part of one member of the family leads to anxiety and problems in the others; they too are thus often in need of support. If the illness is prolonged, it often involves a considerable burden on the family. Many researchers in psychiatric out-patient care have drawn attention to this; Grad's & Sainsbury's publications in the 1960s can be mentioned as an example (e.g. Grad & Sainsbury, 1968). In Finland, Anttinen & Stenij (1974), in their study using a home-care programme as a setting for after-care and rehabilitation of schizophrenic patients, found that the support or treatment of family members was needed in 67 out of the 83 cases where the patient (after discharge from the hospital) moved in with his spouse, parents or children. There were 32 families which included, besides the patient, one or more mentally ill family members.

Such findings imply the importance of family-oriented treatment in schizophrenia in terms of preventive mental health work. This consideration is of particular importance in the case of patients who have established families of their own, and have their own children.

The development of actual family therapy has been influenced by the observation, made by many researchers, that the development of schizophrenia is often associated with problems of the entire family (e.g. Wynne & Singer, 1963; Lidz, Fleck & Cornelison, 1965; Singer & Wynne, 1965; Alanen, 1980) and that the prognosis too is partly dependent on intrafamilial attitudes and changes in the family atmosphere. The latter holds true regardless of aetiology; this has been shown for instance by empirical studies carried out at the London Institute of Psychiatry (Brown, Birley & Wing, 1972; Vaughn & Leff, 1976). It was found in these studies that the chances of the schizophrenic patient, who returns to his family of orientation, not needing rehospitalization is inversely related to the extent of critical and/or emotionally involved communication between the parents and the patient.

Through conjoint family therapy, attended by the patient and other members of his family, such problems may be better solved than through therapeutic work involving the patient alone. In successful family therapy, the family atmosphere and the psychological resources of its members are often observed, in the course of time, to become an important support for the schizophrenic member of the family, assisting his recovery and growth. The families of schizophrenic patients most typically are not rejective toward their patient members, and this (as a rule) constitutes an important element in the state of intrafamilial psychological homeostasis.

Results obtained in family therapy of schizophrenia have been available for over 20 years (e.g. Bowen *et al.*, 1961; Jackson & Weakland, 1961; Esterson, Cooper & Laing, 1965; Scott & Ashworth, 1967; Scott & Montanez, 1972; Alanen & Kinnunen, 1975; Alanen, 1976; Kaufmann, 1976). Most of these reports have dealt with encountering therapy, in which the aim has been in particular the fostering of communication and differentiation between family members. The reports have shared the view that family therapy is a meaningful and, in most cases, an effective mode of treatment.

In recent years the development of family therapy has been largely influenced by a technique developed by the so-called Milano group (Selvini Palazzoli *et al.*, 1978), based on systems theory and teamwork. Therapists working within this framework take active steps to find out in what way the symptoms of the identified patient form part of the family homeostasis and serve to maintain it. When the therapists interpret their views to the family, following a deliberate strategy, they may succeed in transforming the intrafamilial psychological feedback circuits. The study of indicators for this treatment mode, its prerequisites and results lie in the future.

Another currently significant line of development consists of the combination of a directive mode family therapy – often involving educational aims – with drug therapy; its specific object is to prevent rehospitalization. Favourable results obtained by this approach have been reported e.g. by Goldstein *et al.* (1978), Falloon *et al.* (1982) and Leff *et al.* (1982).

The question of the aetiological role of family-dynamic factors in schizophrenia is still the subject of controversy. I myself believe that psychological resistance also plays a role in shaping the attitudes of those who do not ascribe an aetiological significance to them. It is therefore always important to stress that family researchers and family therapists should not see a child's schizophrenia as the patients' fault'. The problems of the parents, as well as those of the children, have their own roots, and attempts should be made to understand both in the same way. Otherwise family therapy has no chance of success. Systems-theoretical ideas tend to accentuate further these lines of thought by placing great emphasis on the active influence exerted by all family members (including the identified patient) on the shared interactional circuit.

Finnish multicentre project for the development of the treatment of new schizophrenics

In Finland a nationwide programme to develop research on and treatment and rehabilitation of schizophrenia was begun in 1981. The purpose of the programme is on the one hand to reduce the amount of chronicization among new schizophrenic patients, on the other to rehabilitate long-term schizophrenics currently under hospital care so as to make their discharge possible. 14 of the 21 mental health districts of the country are actively participating in some of the projects included in the programme. To reach the first objective, a multicentre project for the development of the treatment of new schizophrenic patients was begun in six districts this year. This project was designed partly on the basis of experience gained in a treatment study carried out in Turku in the late 1970s (preliminary results in Alanen *et al.*, 1982*b*; 1983). In the research setting, an attempt will be made to develop treatment practice in a comprehensive way, stimulating psychotherapeutic and family-oriented treatment modes in particular and studying the preconditions and indications for them, and their effect on the patient's prognosis. Drs Viljo Räkköläinen and Raimo K. R. Salokangas are the leaders of this project, the present author is its supervisor. The project has also given rise to collaborative research within the Scandinavian countries (involving three areas in Sweden, one in Norway and one in Denmark, in addition to the six districts in Finland). Cooperation with Scandinavian colleagues has contributed, for instance, to the planning of the research forms used in the study.

The objectives of the multicentre project for the development of the treatment of new schizophrenic patients are the following.

1. The epidemiological objective is the determination of the annual incidence rate of schizophrenia in the districts, located in different parts of the country, at the same time examining background factors of a clinical, demographic, social and family-dynamic nature. As part of the research involves collaboration between the Scandinavian countries, it is of particular interest to see whether the incidence rate is higher for the Finnish than for the Swedish, Norwegian and Danish research areas; there have been certain previous indications that this is the case.
2. It is hoped to encourage comprehensive further development of treatment practice stimulating, in particular, the psychotherapeutic and family-oriented modes of treatment. There are differences in treatment practice and therapeutic resources between different districts, making comparisons between treatment orientations possible.
3. We wish to determine, by means of follow-up evaluations, the success of the therapies, the conditions for success of the various modes of treatment, and the effect of the different treatment modes on prognosis.
4. It is intended to develop useful and effective new approaches to and methods of schizophrenia treatment to serve the needs of the entire Finnish psychiatric health care system.

The patient sample will be gathered during the period extending from 1 March 1983 to 29 February 1984. The study deals with all individuals in the age range 15–44 living in the research districts who come for the first time to a community psychiatric out-patient or in-patient unit for treatment for a schizophrenia-group disorder. In the initial investigation two research forms are used; the one concerns basic social, clinical and psychodynamic data and the other deals with data related to the family. Our diagnostic criteria follow the DSM III classification for schizophrenic and schizophreniform disorders; schizo-affective disorders are also included, in the diagnosis of which Research Diagnostic Criteria according to Spitzer, Endicott & Robins (1978) are used. Follow-up evaluations will be carried out 1, 2 and (hopefully) 5 years after entrance into treatment.

I shall now deal with the lines along which we have planned the development of family-oriented treatment and the various modes of family therapy.

Investigation of the family situation

This forms a basis for the drawing up of a family-oriented treatment plan. Our second research form (the Finnish Form for Schizophrenics' Families, FFSF) is used for this purpose*. An investigation of the family situation is, in our view, necessary in all new cases of schizophrenia. The aim is to find out both the problems present and the extent of positive resources.

The investigation includes basic information on the family; certain family-dynamic assessments primarily related to the year preceding the onset of the illness; and an assessment of the need for treatment of family members and their treatment motivation, which helps in drawing up the treatment plan.

Evaluation of the degree of the patient's inner and outer disengagement from his family of orientation is among the most important psychodynamic assessments. Another group of items, the importance of which I want to emphasize, consists of assessments of the severity of psychological disturbance of the patient's parents and spouse. In our experience the boundary line between disorders of neurotic level and ego disturbance more severe than those occurring in these close relatives is of particular importance in diagnosing the interactional family relationships. Räkköläinen and I have used the term 'transactional defence mechanisms', for 'those defensive functions through which the individual tries to protect himself against anxiety caused by internal or external threats, by drawing on other persons and/or fantasies about them' (Räkköläinen & Alanen, 1982). A tendency to use such defences is particularly common in individuals in whom the disturbance of ego functions is characterized by severe interactional pathology in the form of a pronounced over-dependence on another person or marked tendency to dominate another. Such a

* The form is available from the author.

pathology usually occurs in association with an 'intrapsychic' personality disorder, in particular of a narcissistic, paranoid or dependent type but often also with other severe ego disturbances, including disturbances of psychotic level. The presence of this kind of personality in the parents or spouse of the patient usually necessitates a family-centred treatment approach, at least in the form of a psychological support to the family member in question.

We further evaluate family and other network members' attitudes toward the patient, regarding their capacity for empathic understanding, willingness to provide support for the patient or a rejecting attitude toward him, appreciation or critical attitude towards the patient, and possessive (binding) tendencies inherent in the relationship with him.

The form also includes system-oriented assessments concerning the entire family regarding the stability of the family structure or family adaptibility, family cohesion or closeness (these according to Olson *et al.*, 1979), clarity of communication, the family members' relative power and intrafamilial domination (schismatic and skewed families in the meaning of Lidz, Fleck & Cornelison, 1965), mutual respect and devaluation, the manner of dealing with conflicts, as well as the family's adjustment to the social environment. In our clinical experience, clearly observable deviations from a 'normal state' are common, e.g. regarding the family adaptability and family cohesion in these families (deviations in both directions may also occur simultaneously).

The usefulness of our FFSF in gathering information and in planning treatment can be verified only in the course of our study. I want to emphasize here the function of the form as an instrument for further development and training in the clinical psychiatric work.

Family therapeutic modes of treatment

I shall finally summarize the indications for family-therapeutic modes of treatment, as they have been planned in our project. They are based, above all, on our experience gained so far in Finland (e.g. Alanen, 1976; Alanen *et al.*, 1982*b*).

Encountering and supportive conjoint family therapy of the patient and his family of orientation

This mode of therapy is quite often indicated in the case of young patients and also of older schizophrenic patients living in the childhood home and without an adequate psychological differentiation from it (due to mutual binding interrelationships). A conjoint therapeutic setting helps, often quite effectively, to stimulate the self-expression of even relatively autistic

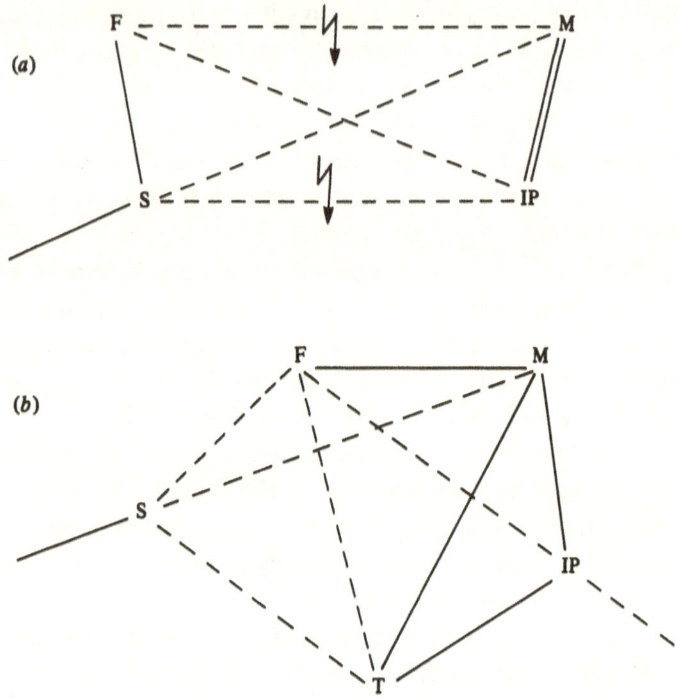

Fig. 2. Encountering and supportive conjoint family therapy, an illustrative case example. (*a*) The family constellation prior to therapy. The family is schismatic: the contact between the parents is diminished and there is fighting (arrow). The mother (M) and the patient child (IP) are bound together symbiotically. There is a well sibling (S) who has a closer relation with the father (F) than with the mother but is, in contrast to the IP, able to form significant relationships outside the family. There is also fighting between the children. (*b*) The family constellation changed by the therapeutic intervention. The family members have formed a relationship with the therapist. This is strongest in the case of M and IP. M has – so to say – switched one of her 'dependency lines' from the patient to the therapist (and is beginning to incorporate some of the therapist's attitudes in her own attitudes towards other family members). IP has more 'space for growth' and is beginning to develop outside contacts. The relationship between F and M has also improved, which has a stabilizing effect in the family network and will strengthen the generation boundaries. S is moving away from the family.

patients and may (if assisted by the therapist) considerably improve the control of aggressions – on the one hand suppressed, on the other explosively vented – leading gradually to more integrated patterns of communication. Separation processes can be supported through measures which help to expand the patient's 'space of growth'. In favourable cases, a gradual process of growth and development takes place in both patient and the family, often accompanied by an increase in positive resources in all the individuals involved.

Such a therapeutic process succeeds best in the case of relatively dynamically 'mobile' but, at the same time, entangled families. A simple example of the way in which the intrafamilial relationships and the state of family interactions can change is shown in the enclosed diagram (Fig. 2).

Another important subgroup consists of families characterized by a chaotic quality, diffuseness of communication or confusion. In these cases, it is especially important for the therapist to aim at enhancement of clarity and enhancement of emotional security.

System-oriented conjoint therapy of the family of orientation

An active system-oriented form of intervention, using the method developed by Selvini Palazzoli *et al.* (1978) is needed most urgently by families characterized by rigidity and/or denial of their conflicts and presenting an intense resistance to change. However, a system-oriented intervention is often also quite effective in cases where an acute schizophrenic psychosis has broken out connected with a conflicting life situation. Specialized training in family therapy is here required and the work should be carried out by a team.

Couple therapy and conjoint therapy of the family of procreation

Couple therapy is often indicated for married or cohabiting patients. Our experience with this mode of therapy has been rather positive and we recommend it also to less experienced family therapists. Its success depends largely on the capacity for empathy on the part of the spouse. In some cases the support provided by the spouse for the patient gains particular prominence, while in others the emphasis is laid on clarifying work on shared problems. The children can best be supported when they are present; it is also important to take their problems into consideration in those cases where they do not participate in therapy.

Support of the family

The investigation of the family situation and the contact thus established at the initial stage provides a good basis for supporting the family and/or its separate members, where indicated. This can be done either in a comprehensive manner, e.g. in a home-care setting with the patient generally present, or separately by meeting specific family members or answering telephone calls from them. The patient should be aware of these activities. Support for family members is particularly indicated when

- another family member besides the patient is individually in need of help or support,

- the family needs support to bear up under the burden caused by the patient's illness and treatment,
- the family serves as an important 'therapeutic channel' (sometimes even the only one) for the patient who is poorly motivated for treatment,
- the patient's individual therapy needs to be supported through contacts with the family.

In the treatment study carried out in the Turku Mental Health District at the end of the 1970s, which I have already referred to (Alanen *et al.*, 1982*b*; 1983; a monograph based on 5-year follow-up is in preparation), individual therapy was more often provided – and with better results – than family therapy. It was noted then that in many cases success in individual therapy was largely dependent on whether a favourable contact had developed with the patient's family members as well. Such contacts are particularly necessary in those cases presenting an indication for individual therapy in which the transactional defence mechanisms used by other family members lead to resistance on the part of the family to the disengagement by the patient from the family. In those cases where conjoint therapy of the family of orientation is the initial mode of therapy, individual therapy of the patient is often subsequently indicated and sustained contacts with family members are sometimes necessary.

In our previous study the most important factor that hampered the provision of family therapy was a lack of sufficient family-therapeutic training. This situation has now changed and the number of trained family therapists available, e.g. in Turku, is higher. Our new Finnish study will provide more information on the indications for family therapy within community psychiatry, on the possibilities of actually providing it and on the results obtained by this therapy.

References

Alanen, Y. O. (1976). On background factors and goals in the family therapy of young schizophrenic patients and their parents. In *Schizophrenia* 75, ed. J. Jörstad & E. Ugelstad. Oslo: Universitetsförlaget.

Alanen, Y. O. (1980). In search of the interactional origin of schizophrenia. The Stanley R. Dean Award Lecture, in *The Family, Evaluation and Treatment*, ed. C. K. Hofling & J. M. Lewis. New York: Brunner/Mazel.

Alanen, Y. O. & Kinnunen, P. (1975). Marriage and the development of schizophrenia. *Psychiatry*, **38**, 346–55.

Alanen, Y. O., Räkköläinen, V. & Laakso, J. (1982*a*). Krankheitsmodelle bei der Schizophrenie und die Bedürfnisangemessenheit der Behandlung. *Nervenarzt*, **53**, 150–3.

Alanen, Y. O., Räkköläinen, V. Laakso, J. & Rasimus, R. (1980). Problems inherent in the study of psychotheraphy of psychoses. In *The Psychotherapy of Schizophrenia*, ed. J. S. Strauss, M. Bowers, T. W. Downey, S. Fleck, S. Jackson & I. Levine. New York: Plenum Publications.

Alanen, Y. O., Räkköläinen, V., Laakso, J., Rasimus, R. & Järvi, R. (1983).

Psychotherapy of schizophrenia in community psychiatry: 2-year follow-up findings and the influence of selective processes in psychotherapeutic treatments. In *Psychosocial Intervention in Schizophrenia*, ed. H. Stierlin, L. C. Wynne & M. Wirsching. Berlin: Springer Verlag.

Alanen, Y. O., Räkköläinen, V., Rasimus, R., Laakso, J. & Järvi, R. (1982*b*). Developing the treatment of schizophrenia in a community-psychiatric setting. A psychotherapeutic and family-centered approach. *Psychiatria Fennica* 1982, 101–20.

Anttinen, E. E. & Stenij, P. (1974). The care and rehabilitation of schizophrenic out-patients with home-care. *Psychiatria Fennica 1974*, 145–54.

Bowen, M., Dysinger, R. H., Brodey, W. M. & Basamania, B. (1961). The family as the unit of study and treatment. *American Journal of Orthopsychiatry*, **31**, 40–86.

Brown, G. W., Birley, J. L. T. & Wing, J. K. (1972). Influence of family life on the course of schizophrenic disorders: a replication. *British Journal of Psychiatry*, **121**, 241–58.

Esterson, A., Cooper, D. G. & Laing, R. D. (1965). Results of family-oriented therapy with hospitalized schizophrenics. *British Medical Journal*, **2**(1965), 1462–5.

Falloon, I. R. H., Boyd, J. L., McGill, C. W., Razani, J., Moss, H. B. & Gilderman, A. M. (1982). Family management in the prevention of exacerbations of schizophrenia: a controlled study. *New England Journal of Medicine*, **306**, 1437–40.

Goldstein, M. J., Rodnick, E. H., Evans, J. R., May, P. R. A. & Steinberg, M. R. (1978). Drug and family therapy in the after-care of acute schizophrenics. *Archives of General Psychiatry*, **35**, 1169–77.

Grad, J. & Sainsbury, P. (1968). The effects that patients have on their families in a community care and a control psychiatric service – a two-year follow-up. *British Journal of Psychiatry*, **114**, 265–78.

Jackson, D. D. & Weakland, J. H. (1961). Conjoint family therapy: some considerations on theory, technique, and results. *Psychiatry*, **24** Suppl. 2, 30–45.

Kaufmann, L. (1976). Long-term family therapy with schizophrenics, in *Schizophrenia* 75, ed. J. Jørstad & E. Ugelstad. Oslo: Universitetsförlaget.

Leff, J., Kuipers, L., Berkowitz, R., Eberlein-Vries, R. & Sturgeon, D. (1982). A controlled trial social intervention in the families of schizophrenic patients. *British Journal of Psychiatry*, **141**, 121–34.

Lidz, T., Fleck, S. & Cornelison, A. R. (1965). *Schizophrenia and the Family*. New York: International University Press.

Olson, D. H., Sprenkle, D. H. & Russell, C. S. (1979). Circumplex model of marital and family systems. I. Cohesion and adaptability dimensions, family types, and clinical applications. *Family Process*, **18**, 3–45.

Räkköläinen, V. & Alanen, Y. O. (1982). On the transactionality of defensive processes. *Psychoanalytic Review*, **9**, 263–72.

Scott, R. D. & Ashworth, P. L. (1967). 'Closure' at the first schizophrenic breakdown: a family study. *British Journal of Medical Psychology*, **40**, 109–45.

Scott, R. D. & Montanez, A. (1972). The nature of tenable and untenable patient-parent relationships and their connection with hospital outcome. In *Psychotherapy of Schizophrenia*, ed. D. Rubinstein & Y. O. Alanen. Amsterdam: Excerpta Medica.

Selvini Palazzoli, M., Boscolo, L., Cecchin, G. & Prata, G. (1978). *Paradox and Counterparadox*. New York: Jason Aronson.

Singer, M. T. & Wynne, L. C. (1965). Thought disorders and family relations of schizophrenics: III–IV. *Archives of General Psychiatry*, **12**, 187–212.

Spitzer, R. L., Endicott, J. & Robins, E. (1978). Research diagnostic criteria: rationale and reliability. *Archives of General Psychiatry*, **35**, 773–82.

Vaughn, C. & Leff, J. (1976). The influence of family and social factors on the course of psychiatric illness. A comparison of schizophrenic and depressed neurotic patients. *British Journal of Psychiatry*, **129**, 125–37.

Wynne, L. C. & Singer, M. T. (1963). Thought disorder and family relations in schizophrenia: I–II. *Archives of General Psychiatry*, **9**, 191–206.

Milieu therapy in the long-term treatment of functional psychoses: needed areas of research

P. VAGLUM AND S. FRIIS

In a time when many people view psychiatric institutions mainly as evils which should be defeated, it might seem unnecessary to examine the present knowledge of milieu therapy and to search for lacunae which should be filled through new scientific activities. Several reasons make it still worthwhile. Firstly, we do not know how to cure all patients with a functional psychosis. New benefits from a more effective milieu therapy would be very welcome. Secondly, in spite of an extensive out-patient service, some patients still have to be treated in in-patient units. We therefore need knowledge about what types of milieu will promote the most favourable outcome for these patients, both in the short and the long run. Thirdly, a large group of psychotic patients will, in the future, be attending day hostels, half-way houses or collectives. Our need for knowledge about the positive and the negative milieu factors in these environments is indisputable. Lastly, all research concerning milieu treatment may be viewed as part of the more general study of the influence of environmental factors upon the course of functional psychoses. It may therefore give us new information about precipitating and possible aetiological factors.

From the title, one would expect this paper to limit itself only to long-term milieu treatment. It does not, and the reason is that to find the optimal duration of milieu therapy for different groups of psychotic patients, we have to be sure that we are studying milieus where the milieu therapy really works. At present it is this last question we are trying to solve.

In modern treatments of functional psychoses, we almost always use a combination of different therapeutic modalities, such as pharmacotherapy, individual psychotherapy, family therapy etc. This paper will deal with milieu therapy as part of such a combination of treatment methods. The possibilities of substituting pharmacotherapy with milieu therapy, will not be discussed.

The idea of a therapeutic milieu

The influence of the social environment upon the course of functional psychoses, has been known for a long time. Since World War II, this knowledge has been further developed through series of observations from hospitals, rehabilitation centres, families and in the community (Wing, 1978). The recognition that the hospital milieu might have noxious effects upon patients through social understimulation, led to very important humanitarian reforms within mental hospitals, and to the development of a variety of alternative forms of out-patient care.

It also led to the idea of creating a social setting where 'bad things' were prevented, where 'good things' might happen, and where pharmacotherapy, occupational therapy and psychotherapy could be used optimally. *Milieu treatment* became a broad concept meaning a specialized environment designed to fulfil such general purposes (Gunderson, 1978). In many countries, this idea became very popular. Most wards with a minimum of self respect would claim to offer milieu treatment. Stanton's (1962) statement 'There is no patient 'untreated' by his environment, only patients 'treated' well or ill' was widely accepted. Consequently, the whole staff became milieu therapists, whether they wanted it or not. Looking back, it is not difficult to see that such a situation could easily compromise the milieu treatment method, ending up with vague concepts and a large distance between ideals and realities (Vaglum *et al.*, 1982).

One trend in the milieu treatment movement has limited itself mostly to prevent social over- or understimulation, and to create an adequate social context for the practice of more traditional treatment methods. Another trend has been more ambitious, that of trying to use the milieu as a treatment method of its own: as a *milieu therapy*. The pioneers of the therapeutic community movement (Main, 1946; Jones *et al.*, 1952; Wilmer, 1958) (and later, in part, the behaviour treatment movement) claimed that it would be possible to design a social structure and a set of patient and staff activities which would promote specific emotional and learning experiences which would change the behaviour and the personality of the patients in specific directions.

The theory and practice of the therapeutic community has influenced the organization and activities of many psychiatric institutions in many countries. Some have tried to develop a 'therapeutic community proper' (Clark, 1977), others have used elements or modifications from the therapeutic community. Because milieu treatment and the therapeutic community were for a long time looked upon as a panacea which was good for all patients, patients with acute and chronic functional psychoses have also been exposed to these forms of treatment. What have we learnt about the suitability of milieu therapy after an encounter of nearly 40 years between the ideas of a therapeutic milieu and the obstinate reality? Three questions are particularly important:

1. Does milieu treatment work?
2. How do we measure the therapeutic variables of treatment milieus?
3. What are the therapeutic characteristics of therapeutic milieus?

Does milieu treatment work?

No conclusive evidence has been produced up to now on whether milieu treatment works, but substantial progress has been made during the last 10 years. The question of whether it works for schizophrenic patients can now be answered with 'sometimes yes, sometimes no'. Why it varies, however, we do not know. May & Simpson (1980) found, in their extensive and highly critical review of the experimental studies of in-patient milieu treatment, 14 studies with positive results, 9 with doubtful positive and 9 with negative results. All eight studies which evaluated the effect of out-patient after-care and rehabilitation programmes showed positive results. Several studies comparing milieu treatment and drug treatment have also found that unmedicated patients in specially designed milieu treatment, can do as well as medicated patients. Other studies have shown that the need for (or use of) medication may be reduced in an intensively working milieu therapy unit (Mosher, 1980). These findings give additional support to the notion that milieu therapy does influence the course of functional psychoses and should be viewed as a therapy of its own.

There are many weaknesses in these experimental and quasi-experimental studies. One serious problem, which constitutes one of the special problems in milieu therapy research (Dalgard *et al.*, 1983), is the use of designs in which one milieu treatment programme is compared with another. As we still do not know exactly which milieu characteristics are therapeutic (or antitherapeutic), it is almost impossible to know whether the milieus of the wards compared, really were significantly different in regard to the important variables. By and large, up to now the design of the milieu therapy programmes has *not* been accomplished by identifying and putting together a few milieu factors with a known therapeutic effect, later adding new factors only if they had been proved to be therapeutic. Instead, milieu programmes have usually been designed as complex programmes with a large set of structural and behavioural variables. These have been selected partly on the basis of common sense, partly on the basis of theoretical thinking and clinical experience of the effect of large and small groups. Rarely have they been selected because they were known to have a specific therapeutic impact upon the course of functional psychoses. In spite of relatively extensive prescriptions of how to structure a milieu therapeutic ward and its activities, even wards that claim to be a therapeutic community proper, may vary extensively on a lot of variables (Clark, 1977). To understand the clinical and research implications of this variation, we need to study whether single or clusters of milieu variables influence the outcome more than others.

How do we measure the therapeutic variables of treatment milieus?

Over the past 15 years, some progress has been made in research on identifying the therapeutic variables of the milieu. Initially, this research was mostly concerned with the relationship between structural variables and in-patient behaviour. Since in-patient adjustment seemed to be poorly related to adaptation in the community, the research has lately been concentrated on finding milieu characteristics which are correlated to the course after discharge.

Two types of milieu variables have been studied: behavioural and apprehensive. To know exactly what staff and patients are doing on a behavioural level, is undoubtedly important. Paul & Lentz (1977) have therefore made an important contribution to the study of treatment milieus for chronic schizophrenic patients by developing the Staff Resident Interaction Chronograph (SRIC). Its value for studying milieus for a non-chronic population, is still to be established.

Even if it is important to describe the organizational structure of wards exactly and to measure staff and patient behaviour, we obviously need additional measures. From a theoretical point of view, there is an important intervening variable between behaviour and its impact on the patients' psychopathological conditions: the patients' apprehension of the behaviour. This has also been clearly demonstrated by life event research; the person's apprehension of the event is more important than what happened in practice. Theoretically, it may be that milieus that are meant to be similar, still may be perceived as different by the patients. It may also be that milieus which are both meant and perceived to be different from the staff's point of view, still are perceived as being rather similar by the patients. This is demonstrated in a comparison of therapeutic communities and traditional wards by Steiner, Haldipur & Stack (1982).

A reliable and valid instrument for measuring the staff's and the patients' perception of the milieu was therefore urgently needed. Moos & Houts (1968) brought this field a significant step forward by their construction of the Ward Atmosphere Scale (WAS). This scale measures how the patient and the staff group perceive the level of involvement, support, spontaneity, autonomy, practical orientation, personal problem orientation, anger and aggression, order and organization (structure and predictability), programme clarity and staff control. It has proved to have satisfactory internal consistency and inter-rater reliability (Moos, 1974; Friis, 1984). The WAS-scores have a high stability over months and are sensitive to planned, structural changes of ward milieus (Friis, 1981*a*; Pierce, Trickett & Moos, 1972). National reference groups of wards have been made in the USA and, lately, in Norway (Friis, 1981*b*). WAS has been translated into several languages, and a comparison of the results from four different countries indicates that the scale has excellent cross-cultural properties (Friis, 1984). As staff's WAS-scores may not give very reliable measures of the patients' perception of the same ward (Friis, 1984), the WAS-scores ought to be calculated for patients and staff members separately. The course of the psychiatric conditions is probably more closely associated with the patients' perceptions than with the staff's perceptions of the milieu. It is therefore a highly questionable procedure to use the pooled staff and patient scores as a measure of the ward atmosphere.

What are the therapeutic characteristics of therapeutic milieus?

For *chronic schizophrenic* patients, Mosher (1980) and May & Simpson (1980) conclude in their reviews that such patients seem to respond best to an in-patient milieu which is very structured, highly organized and with high expectations and which is orientated towards specific behaviour change, followed by an extensive and differentiated out-patient care. Paul & Lentz (1977) obtained remarkably good results in such a behaviour orientated (token economy) programme.

Mosher (1980) and Gunderson (1980) have recently made extensive reviews of studies concerning the therapeutic factors in the treatment of *acute schizophrenia*. They conclude that acute schizophrenic patients have been found to recover best in highly staffed, accepting, supportive, stimulus decreasing, relatively long-stay (3–5 months) environments in which psychosocial interventions are viewed positively. In addition, four milieu characteristics have been found to be associated with better post-hospital psychosocial adjustment: (*a*) small size (< 10 beds), (*b*) positive staff expectations, (*c*) line staff's active involvement in the treatment and decision making, and (*d*) a practical down-to-earth problem-solving attitude.

How are such milieus perceived by the patients? Based upon the 1980 reviews by Mosher and Gunderson and the theoretical considerations of Kernberg (1976), one would expect such milieus to be characterized (in

WAS-terms) by a high level of support, practical orientation, order and organization (structure and predictability) and programme clarity, and by a low level of anger and aggression. Unfortunately, WAS has up to now been used only in a few investigations of post-hospital outcome. The results so far are not conclusive.

Moos & Schwartz (1972) and Moos, Shelton & Petty (1973) have reported two studies from large Veterans Administration (VA) hospitals in the USA. The studies did not, however, control for pre- and post-discharge variables, and possible differential effects on different types of patients were not examined.

Klass, Growe & Strizich (1977) managed to eliminate some of these methodological problems in their study of wards for mainly psychotic (mostly chronic schizophrenic) patients. They found that the community tenure rate was strongly negatively correlated with the perceived level of anger and aggression (patients and staff), and positively correlated with the level of order and organization (staff).

Both in the patient and staff group, there was a strong, negative correlation between anger and aggression and order and organization. In this study, there was no difference between the wards on support and practical orientation. The relationship between these variables and the outcome, could therefore not be examined.

The possible importance of the level of anger and aggression and order and organization was supported by a study from our institute (Friis, 1984). Patients from twelve Norwegian wards for mainly psychotic patients were asked to answer both WAS and a questionnaire concerning their appreciation of their ward. The patients' appreciation was strongly positively correlated with the perceived level of support, practical orientation and order and organization, and negatively with the level of anger and aggression at the ward. Wards with less than 16 patients were found to be closer to this presumed beneficial WAS-profile than wards with more than 16 patients.

These investigations only permit suggestions. The relationship between good outcome and both a high level of order and organization and a low level of anger and aggression seems to be most convincingly documented. The evidence seems also to suggest that a high level of support and practical orientation may be important.

The finding that a low degree of anger and aggression may be related to a positive outcome, is important for two reasons. This is parallel to the finding from studies of family milieus which shows that the degree of aggression in the family is strongly correlated to psychotic relapses (Leff *et al.*, 1982). It also questions the idea of the therapeutic community proper, that all affects should be expressed openly. Rapoport (1960) found that only 25% of the psychotic patients, in contrast to 77% of the neurotic patients, improved in the therapeutic community of Belmont.

New questions – needed research

Identification of the profile of at least four ward atmosphere variables characterizing a milieu expected to have a beneficial effect upon schizophrenic patients, opens up the possibilities of a variety of new studies. Firstly, we need several attempts to replicate these findings as well as new *outcome studies* looking for other milieu variables. In such studies, it will be necessary to use more valid outcome variables than most of the milieu therapy studies have been using up to now (drop-out rate, release rate, community tenure). Schizophrenic patients treated in wards with significantly different WAS-profiles should be followed through their stay as in-patients and for several years afterwards on such variables as psychopathology, social functioning, quality of life, relationships, attitudes to their psychosis, and exposure to all forms of out-patient treatment. In the most chronic population, the applicability of WAS is limited because too many patients will be incapable of answering the questions. For the studies of the milieu therapy of these populations, the SRIC seems to be a very useful alternative.

Another group of studies has to try to answer the question of how we should manage to develop and maintain a therapeutic milieu perceived by the patients as high in order and organization, support and practical orientation, and low in anger and aggression? What are the combinations of philosophical, structural and behavioural variables which result in such a WAS-profile? It is apparently not enough to fulfil the four criteria that Gunderson (1980) found to be characteristic of three successful milieu therapy programmes.

> First, all of the units had a high staff/patient ratio and were relatively small units. The staff members were predominantly youthful contemporaries of the patients. Second, there was a distribution of responsibility among all staff members, and the patients were believed capable of assuming social responsibility. Third, all three units viewed psychosis as a process to be understood, lived through and accepted. Fourth, all of the units were attempting something iconoclastic, i.e. a mode of therapy at variance with the norms of treatment. Gunderson (1980)

This is illustrated by a recent study of Lehman *et al.* (1982) which compared the outcome of two groups of first admission patients (40–50%

psychotic), one treated in a medically oriented ward and one in a therapeutic community *in statu nascendi.* The therapeutic community ward fulfilled all of the four criteria mentioned by Gunderson, but there was still no difference between the wards in the outcome.

Looking at the WAS-findings it is, however, doubtful whether the wards were sufficiently different on the most important milieu variables. The therapeutic community was perceived by patients and staff collectively as higher on practical orientation (probably beneficial), higher on anger and aggression (probably detrimental), lower on order and organization (probably detrimental), and equal on support. Because the WAS-scores were calculated from the pooled scores of patients and staff (Lehman & Ritzler, 1976), it is not possible to know whether the patients perceived the wards as being significantly different in regard to the most important four WAS-variables. It is our experience that ideologically different wards are perceived to be less different by the patients than by the staff. The findings show, however, that even if Gunderson's four criteria are fulfilled, a therapeutic community ward may have both a partly negative WAS-profile and a treatment outcome which is not better than a traditional, medically oriented ward. Consequently, it is necessary to look for other and possibly more influential milieu characteristics.

One of the central therapeutic tools of the milieu treatment of both acute and chronic schizophrenic patients, has been the use of large and small groups of different kinds. It is therefore highly surprising to find that in most of the milieu therapy studies, the description of the quality and quantity of group exposure, and the relative amount of group and individual therapy, is either neglected or rather vague. Also in the comparisons between programmes, the group variable is usually neglected.

As to the *quantity of group exposure*, the negative experiences with a therapeutic community model of Letemendia, Harris & Williams (1967), Spadoni & Smith (1969) and van Putten (1973) seem to come from wards with a high amount of group exposure, and with virtually no individual psychotherapy or formation of one-to-one relationships. The positive experiences of Madew, Singer & Macindoe (1966), Denber, Turns & Seeman (1968) and Jeffrey, Kleban & Papernik (1976) seem to come from programmes with the opposite profile. Vaglum & Bøe (unpublished data) found that the outcome after discharge from a therapeutic community was significantly worsened in the group of schizophrenics when the amount of group exposure was increased from 13 to 23 hours per week. When the patients at follow-up were asked to describe factors which they thought to be therapeutic or not, they first of all emphasized a lack of good one-to-one relationships as the most antitherapeutic factor (Vaglum & Bøe 1981).

As to the *quality of group work* in therapeutic milieus, we are also too short of knowledge. How does one conduct large and small groups in a ward or a day centre with mainly psychotic patients? S. Karterud (personal communication) recently found in a study from our institute, that the quality of the living/learning groups of three therapeutic community wards varied a great deal. In some groups it was sometimes impossible to develop the group as a psychological reality at all when the percentage of psychotic patients was high. We urgently need research directed to the question of which factors promote or inhibit therapeutic group processes in wards for different types of psychotic patients. In such research, both the amount and quality of group work should be described as thoroughly as possible.

In our further search for therapeutic milieu variables and their degree of inter-relatedness, both *explorative, descriptive and experimental designs* should be used. By comparing wards which are meant to be similar, but still have different WAS-profiles, and by comparing wards which are meant to be different and either have different or similar WAS-profiles, it should be possible to identify new clusters of important milieu factors. Their influence upon the course of the psychoses should then be examined further in outcome studies. Experimental and quasi-experimental intensive designs of the AB or ABA type, will make it possible to test what consequences operationally defined alterations in a milieu therapy programme might have on the patients' WAS-scores. In such a study at our institute, we reduced the amount of group exposure by two-thirds in a therapeutic community proper, with mainly acute psychotic patients. The therapeutic philosophy was also changed from a purely group-oriented to a more individual-oriented type. The number of patients was also reduced from 30 to 20. The patients' score on three of the four crucial WAS-variables mentioned earlier, altered significantly in a favourable direction. So did the patients' appreciation of the milieu (Vaglum, Friis & Karterud, unpublished data).

In all future studies, it will also be necessary to consider the percentage of *psychotic patients* in the programmes. Friis (1984) found that there was a significant difference in WAS-profiles between wards with mainly psychotic patients and wards with mainly non-psychotic patients.

What is the best milieu for different types of psychotic patients?

Up to now, most of the milieu research has been concentrated on the question whether a programme or single milieu characteristic will work at all. The recent development of the classification of patients (DSM III, ICD 9) and of ward milieus, has increased the possibility of looking for different therapeutic processes and effects within the group of psychotic patients. McGlashan & Levy (1977) have, for instance, underlined that the psychotic patients differ in the process of recovery; some recover mostly by sealing over, others mostly by integrating. Heim *et al.* (1975) observed in a study from Schlössli that some schizophrenic patients actively participated in the therapeutic community, while others did not. Obviously, there are such great differences within and between the group of acute and chronic schizophrenic patients, that one should search continuously for subgroups which need special milieus.

Every single psychotic patient might also need different milieus at different points of time after his breakdown. It might very well be that what is a good milieu the first 6 weeks, may be an indifferent milieu the next 18 weeks, and a disaster during the following months and years. Longitudinal studies, both of a case study type and with relatively small groups of patients, may give us new ideas about how long, how flexible and how differentiated programmes of milieu therapy within and outside psychiatric institutions should be. Such studies will also give valuable information about the degree of inter-relation between milieu variables and the practice of individual psychotherapy, family therapy and group therapy.

Conclusion

In spite of 40 years of milieu treatment, we still do not know enough about how to develop and maintain an optimal milieu therapy for patients with functional psychoses. Milieu therapy research has up to now been able to demonstrate that such therapy sometimes works and sometimes does not. During the recent years, a cluster of milieu characteristics which should be expected to constitute a more optimal therapeutic milieu, has emerged. Outcome seems to be correlated to the patients' perception of the milieu. A favourably perceived milieu is supposed to be characterized by a combination of a high level of order and organization, practical orientation and support, and a low level of anger and aggression. Such a profile may be promoted by a high staff/patient ratio, a relatively small number of patients, a distribution of responsibilities and decision-making power combined with clear roles and leadership, and last, but not least, an adequate quantity and quality of group work and individual therapy. The challenge to clinicians and the researchers is now to carry out such milieu therapy in practice, and over and over again evaluate whether it works, under what conditions, for how long, and for whom. The field is still wide open.

References

Clark, D. H. (1977). The therapeutic community. *British Journal of Psychiatry*, **131**, 553–64.

Dalgard, O. S., Friis, S., Sørensen, T. & Vaglum, P. (1983). Special problems in evaluation of milieu therapy. In *Methodology in Evaluation of Psychiatric Treatment*, ed. T. Helgason, pp. 137–48. Cambridge University Press.

Denber, H., Turns, D. & Seeman, M. (1968). The therapeutic community: nine years after. *Psychiatric Quarterly*, **42**, 531–7.

Friis, S. (1981*a*). From enthusiasm to resignation in a therapeutic community: a process evaluation. *Journal of Oslo City Hospitals*, **31**, 51–4.

Friis, S. (1981*b*). Hva slags postatmosfære er terapeutisk for psykotiske pasienter? *Tidsskrift for den norske lægeforening*, **101**, 848–52.

Friis, S. (1984). *The Ward Atmosphere. A crucial dimension of inpatient settings*. Akad. diss. Oslo University.

Gunderson, J. G. (1978). Defining the therapeutic processes in psychiatric milieus. *Psychiatry*, **41**, 327–35.

Gunderson, J. G. (1980). A reevaluation of milieu therapy for nonchronic schizophrenic patients. *Schizophrenia Bulletin*, **6**, 64–9.

Heim, E., Johnsen, E., Lilienfeld, C., Stauffacher, H. & Wirs, P. (1975). Application of the principles of the therapeutic community with the participation of schizophrenics. In *Schizophrenia 75*, ed. J. Jørstad & E. Ugelstad, pp. 327–46. Oslo: Universitetsforlaget.

Jeffrey, W. D., Kleban, C. H. & Papernik, D. S. (1976). Schizophrenia: treatment in therapeutic community. *New York State Journal of Medicine*, **76**, 384–90.

Jones, M., Baker, A., Freeman, T., Merry, J., Pomryn, B. A., Sandler, J. & Tuxford, J. (1952). *Social Psychiatry. A Study of Therapeutic Communities*. London: Tavistock Publications.

Kernberg, O. F. (1976). *Object Relation Theory and Clinical Psychoanalysis*. Chapter IX: Toward an integrative theory of hospital treatment, pp. 241–75. New York: J. Aronson.

Klass, D. G., Growe, A. & Strizich, M. (1977). Ward treatment milieu and post-hospital functioning. *Archives of General Psychiatry*, **34**, 1047–52.

Leff, J., Kuipers, L., Berkowitz, R., Eberlein Vries, R. & Sturgeon, D. (1982). A controlled trial of social intervention in the families of schizophrenic patients. *British Journal of Psychiatry*, **141**, 121–34.

Lehman, A. & Ritzler, B. (1976). The therapeutic community inpatient ward: does it really work? *Comprehensive Psychiatry*, **17**, 755–61.

Lehman, A., Strauss, J. S., Ritzler, B., Kohes, R. F., Harder, D. W. & Gift, T. E. (1982). First admission psychiatric ward milieu. *Archives of General Psychiatry*, **39**, 1293–8.

Letemendia, F. J. J., Harris, A. D. & Willems, P. J. A. (1967). The clinical effects on a population of chronic schizophrenic patients of administrative changes in hospital. *British Journal of Psychiatry*, **113**, 959–71.

McGlashan, T. & Levy, S. (1977). Sealing-over in a therapeutic community. *Psychiatry*, **40**, 55–65.

Madew, L., Singer, G. & Macindoe, I. (1966). Treatment and rehabilitation in the therapeutic community: a progress report. *The Medical Journal of Australia*, **1**, 1112–14.

Main, T. (1946). The hospital as a therapeutic institution. *Bulletin of Menninger Clinic*, **10**, 66–70.

May, P. & Simpson, G. (1980). Schizophrenia: evaluation of treatment methods. In *Comprehensive Textbook of Psychiatry*, ed. H. Kaplan, A. Freedman & B. Saddock, pp. 1240–51. Baltimore: Williams & Wilkins.

Moos, R. (1974). *Ward Atmosphere Scale Manual*. Palo Alto, Cal.: Consulting Psychologists Press Inc.

Moos, R. & Houts, P. (1968). The assessment of the social atmosphere of psychiatric wards. *Journal of Abnormal Psychology*, **73**, 595–604.

Moos, R. & Schwartz, J. (1972). Treatment environment and treatment outcome. *Journal of Nervous and Mental Disease*, **154**, 264–75.

Moos, R., Shelton, R. & Petty, C. (1973). Perceived ward climate and treatment outcome. *Journal of Abnormal Psychology*, **82**, 291–8.

Mosher, L. (1980). Schizophrenia: recent research trends. In *Comprehensive Textbook of Psychiatry*, ed. H. Kaplan, A. Freedman & B. Saddock, pp. 1275–87. Baltimore: Williams & Wilkins.

Paul, G. & Lentz, R. (1977). *Psychosocial Treatment of Chronic Mental Patients*. London: Harvard University Press.

Pierce, W., Trickett, E. J. & Moos, R. H. (1972). Changing ward atmosphere through staff discussion of the perceived ward environment. *Archives of General Psychiatry*, **26**, 35–41.

Rapoport, R. N. (1960). *Community as Doctor*. London: Tavistock Publications, Charles C. Thomas.

Spadoni, A. & Smith, J. (1969). Milieu therapy in schizophrenia: a negative result. *Archives of General Psychiatry*, **20**, 547–51.

Stanton, A. H. (1962). Foreword. In *Ego and Milieu*. J. Cumming & E. Cumming. New York: Atherton Press.

Steiner, H., Haldipur, C. V. & Stack, L. C. (1982). The acute admission ward as a therapeutic community. *American Journal of Psychiatry*, **139**, 897–901.

Vaglum, P. & Bøe, L. (1981). What was helpful and what was harmful? Patients evaluate the process of recovery in a therapeutic community. *Journal of Oslo City Hospitals*, **31**, 55–8.

Vaglum, P., Friis, S., Jørstad, J., Karterud, S. & Lorentzen, S. (1982). From a panacea to a special treatment method. *International Journal of Therapeutic Communities*, **1**, 24–32.

van Putten, T. (1973). Milieu therapy: contraindications? *Archives of General Psychiatry*, **29**, 640–3.

Wilmer, H. (1958). *Social Psychiatry in Action*. Springfield: Charles C. Thomas.

Wing, J. K. (1978). The social context of schizophrenia. *American Journal of Psychiatry*, **135**, 1333–9.

Long-term treatment of functional psychosis with neuroleptics

R. ÖHMAN AND R. AXELSSON

In many countries the period around 1950 was one in which preparations for great changes were being made within the big mental hospitals. These carried, as they largely do now, the major part of the burden of providing care to those chronically ill with psychotic disorders. Occupational rehabilitation programmes and the active resocialization of severely ill patients were introduced as fundamental parts of open-door policies. There was an increasing improvement in economic and personnel resources above the thresholds necessary simply for the provision of shelter and protection.

The qualities and organization of psychiatric rehabilitation programmes that were known before the drug era have been forgotten and rediscovered several times. The absence of effective modes of drug treatment itself leads to an evaluation of alternative methods of treatment. The importance of a continuous rehabilitation process for chronic psychotics which includes contact with work and family and with medical supervision has been emphasized and clearly demonstrated. The relative ineffectiveness of psychoanalytically oriented therapies has become evident. The value of integrated supportive psychotherapeutic strategies to strengthen motivation, independence and resistance to psychotic breakthrough is also generally accepted (May, 1968; Wing & Brown, 1970; Brown, Birley & Wing, 1972).

The advent of the specific psychopharmacological agents, especially neuroleptics, has greatly increased the possibilities open to mental health systems in the organization of much more efficient rehabilitation programmes for chronic psychoses. The unique properties of the drugs to reduce symptoms of schizophrenic psychosis have been determinant in the further development of our treatment programmes.

Over the last 30 years with neuroleptics, we have, nevertheless, forgotten much about the natural course of chronic psychoses and principles of care. We have been disappointed that neuroleptics do not offer total cure but only relief and at times the dependency of the effect we need on other therapeutic programmes has been neglected. The consequent negative attitude to drugs among laymen and even paramedical staff has led to unrealistic expectations over alternative treatment programmes, none of which is new; they are already ranked as more or less complementary measures in the total organization of mental health care of chronic psychoses.

It is necessary to adopt a historical perspective when trying to evaluate today's therapeutic principles and when designing new strategies for the treatment of chronic psychosis and research in the field.

Patients subject to long-term treatment with neuroleptic drugs are largely suffering from schizophrenic psychosis with florid symptomatology. If offered insufficient medication, they have a tendency to severe relapse which may not only be extremely painful as they return to a world of anxiety, incapacity and delusions, but the possibility of their social and occupational rehabilitation may be severely damaged and their association to family and work-mates undermined. Relapses are periods of high risk for suicide attempts and are also a burden on the mental health care system from an economic point of view, directing attention and resources to a tedious recycling process instead of towards preventive and rehabilitation measures. If the treatment with neuroleptic drugs has proved efficient in ameliorating psychiatric symptomatology in the individual patient, the professional monitoring of the long-term treatment is a most rewarding task.

It will test the psychiatrist's patience and capacity to create a constructive psychological understanding with the patient. Treatment, that may last for several years, will involve a number of practical and ethical problems concerning consent, side-effects of the drug, family reactions etc., as well as more cost–benefit aspects. Finally, it is necessary that the physician responsible for the treatment develops an expertise in the field of clinical pharmacology of neuroleptic drugs.

The general clinical principles concerning the long-term treatment with neuroleptic drugs of patients suffering from chronic psychoses are well established among the medical profession. The detail, however, may be subject to large variations in such choices as the type and dose of the primary drug, e.g. low or high dose type of phenothiazines or butyrophenones, or preference for oral versus depot preparations. The effectiveness of neuroleptics, if administered adequately, to prevent relapses into psychotic episodes has been shown beyond doubt (Goldberg, Klerman &

Cole, 1965; Davis, 1975; Hogarty, Goldberg, Schooler & Ulrich, 1974; Wistedt, 1981). In the light of 30 years of clinical use, marketed neuroleptics must be regarded as safe drugs accepting that there is an array of side effects, which may be the price to pay for effective treatment. However, when examining goals for future research in the area, specific problems deserve further discussion.

It is the patient who is going to benefit but also to suffer from our efforts to arrest a pathological process in order to normalize behaviour and enable optimal social adaptation. His or her understanding or acceptance of psychopathology may vary and is often absent. Our persuasion or enforcement of treatment must rest on careful diagnostic work and the conviction that long-term treatment with neuroleptics is mandatory, in view of the patient's type and intensity of psychotic symptomatology. The present diagnostic systems need further development to provide efficient tools for prospective studies on the outcome of alternative treatment programmes based on the use of neuroleptics. The multiaxial diagnostic systems, first described by Essen-Möller, and now developed for routine clinical use (DSM III) may provide such information. It should also be mentioned, that schizophrenic psychosis seemingly changes in appearance over time. Modern society tends to hide and partially adapt to psychotic individuals in social rehabilitation programmes and sheltered jobs. Adequate psychiatric intervention is often very late or neglected. The long-term consequence deserves specific attention, both from a psychiatric and an economic point of view. It is also questionable whether decentralized psychiatric services will have the resources necessary for observation and diagnosis or will give the priority to such seemingly cared-for individuals who can not advocate their needs. The tremendous break-through made by chlorpromazine and haloperidol was followed by an avalanche of new neuroleptic compounds. Molecular manipulations of the parent neuroleptics have taught us a lot about the ground rules for their action and pharmacokinetics. From a clinical point of view, thioridazine, levopromazine, perphenazine and phimozide have contributed somewhat different neuroleptic profiles of action. Depot-preparations have become important particularly for the long-term management of patients with a low degree of motivation to treatment. Pimozide, clozapine and benzamides, now being introduced, have, however, from a pharmacological point of view a receptor antagonist profile, different from previous drugs. Clinical studies should be initiated to see if their efficiency in long-term treatment differs from that of conventional drugs. Special attention should also be paid to the development of late side effects which may show a novel pattern.

In the near future, new drugs with a neuroleptic type of action will be introduced. Presynaptic dopamine agonists and drugs interfering with the transport of dopamine and its precursors offer such properties. Manipulation of the biosynthesis of receptor protein suggests other possible routes to the development of new drugs with antipsychotic effects.

During recent years much effort has been devoted to the development of so called treatment programmes. Detailed regulations covering the treatment of psychiatric disorders imply a grotesque over-simplication of the task. The treatment – for example the long-term treatment with neuroleptics of chronic psychosis – is a truly unique interaction process where both the patient and the physician are unique personalities. The behaviour of a drug within the individual is also unique showing 10–50 fold variation in essential pharmacokinetics and pharmacodynamics. Finally, the patient's environment of personal support from psychiatry, family and work always represents a unique constellation.

What are needed are ground rules covering desirable routines for continuity, drug monitoring by serum concentration, formal evaluation of effect and side effects and the personal responsibilities of staff for a particular patient under long-term treatment. The overall responsibility for paramedical personnel continuously to motivate the patient to receive treatment once it has proved to be effective is of particular importance. The patient is the one to pay the price for failure and the contribution of all involved must be concerted. Some phases of treatment may need the support of a realistic legislation that in a true sense guards the patient's rights.

Drug-licensing authorities, and therefore also the pharmaceutical companies providing neuroleptic drugs, direct tremendous efforts to the study of side effects such as tardive dyskinesias which are the subject of much concern. There is a need for a great deal of research to illuminate the biological mechanism underlying these phenomena. For a long time to come, they cannot be avoided because of the central role of neuroleptics in the treatment of psychotic states. Specific attention must be directed to the development of predictive models to study different types of drugs and their metabolites, and their tendency to induce tardive dyskinesias. Owing to their finally irreversible nature it is essential to evaluate the significance of these side effects when considering the risks of long-term treatment. Otherwise, our long-term experience with neuroleptics leads us to regard them as safe (Klawans, Goetz & Perlik, 1980). Toxic reactions and other medically important phenomena are seldomly seen. For the patient, however, quite other problems come into focus. He will not worry much over a dry mouth, slightly raised levels of liver transaminases, a remote risk of glaucoma or possible increase of risk for epileptic seizures. However, excessive weight gain, sexual disturbances, feelings of psychological unease and lack of incentive are of great significance to the patient. Much too little attention has been devoted to such phenomena which are central to the patient and often determining in governing compliance to the offered drug regimen.

The explosion of the neurosciences during the 1970s will affect and change the role of the psychiatrist in the future and produce new demands. The long-term treatment of functional psychosis with neuroleptics will also change. Cerebral blood flow studies, NMR, refined techniques for evoked potentials, neuroendocrine studies, functional receptor studies *in vivo* may provide variables used in diagnostic work together with conventional psychiatric methodology for classification and decision on therapeutic strategies.

New families of antipsychotic drugs will emerge, hopefully more efficient in relation to side effects (Carlsson, 1978). Monitoring antipsychotic treatment through serum levels of active drug will soon be the rule since they safeguard against over- and undertreatment from a pharmacokinetic perspective (Axelsson & Mårtensson, 1976). New techniques seem to be developing, whereby the individual's sensitivity to drugs can be illustrated and the optimum serum drug levels predicted (Öhman & Axelsson, 1980).

The increasing problems in funding mental health programmes will also demand that the psychiatrist takes an active part in the economic evaluation of treatment efforts. This is not a task for the economist administrator with no possibility of fully understanding the medical decisions underlying our obligation to support the individual patient in an individual way (and not in a streamlined, normalized treatment programme). The area is of high priority for research. The long-term treatment of psychosis with neuroleptic drugs with high preventive capacity – so costly if mismanaged – is a primary target for such studies.

Acknowledgement

The study was performed with financial support from the Swedish Medical Research Council, project B84-21X-4803-9A.

References

Axelsson, R. & Mårtensson, E. (1976). Serum concentration and elimination from serum of thioridazine in psychiatric patients. *Current Therapeutic Research*, **19**, 396–411.

Brown, G. W., Birley, J. L. T. & Wing, J. K. (1972). Influence of family life on the course of schizophrenia disorders: a replication. *British Journal of Psychiatry*, **121**, 241–58.

Carlsson, A. (1978). Antipsychotic drugs, neurotransmitters and schizophrenia. *American Journal of Psychiatry*, **135**, 164–73.

Davis, J. M. (1975). Clinical pharmacology and the prescription of psychotropic medication. *Pharmacopsychiatria*, **8**, 332–9.

Goldberg, S. C., Klerman, G. L. & Cole, J. O. (1965). Changes in schizophrenic psychopathology and ward behaviour as a function of phenothiazine treatment. *British Journal of Psychiatry*, **111**, 120–33.

Hogarty, G. E., Goldberg, S. C., Schooler, N. R. & Ulrich, R. F. (1974). Drug and sociotherapy in the aftercare of schizophrenic patients. *Archives of General Psychiatry*, **31**, 603–8.

Klawans, H. L., Goetz, C. G. & Perlik, S. (1980). Tardive dyskinesia; reviews and update. *American Journal of Psychiatry*, **137**, 900–8.

May, P. R. A. (1968). *Treatment of schizophrenia*. New York: Science House.

Öhman, R. & Axelsson, R. (1980). Prolactin response to neuroleptics, clinical and theoretical implications. *Journal of Neural Transmission*, Suppl. 17, 1–75.

Wing, J. K. & Brown, G. W. (1970). *Institutionalism and schizophrenia*. London: Cambridge University Press.

Wistedt, B. (1981). A depot neuroleptic withdrawal study. *Acta Psychiatrica Scandinavica*, **64**, 65–84.

Lithium and prophylaxis in manic-depressive illness

P. VESTERGAARD

Introduction

The benefits for manic-depressive patients of long-term lithium treatment are well established. Lithium is unrivalled for episode prevention in bipolar illness (Schou, 1979*a*) and is at least as effective as other treatments for prevention in unipolar illness (Schou, 1979*b*). Also the risks and inconveniences of long-term lithium treatment are well described and understood (Vestergaard, 1983*a*, *b*). Some important problems, however, remain unsolved; one is that lithium does not effectively prevent episode recurrence in *all* patients with manic-depressive illness. Another is that, even when lithium exerts effective prophylaxis, some patients do not adhere to the treatment, this is either because they do not tolerate lithium or because they do not accept the treatment regimen. The first problem may be dealt with in two ways: one is to examine variables which predict good response to lithium treatment; the other is to search for alternative or additional treatments which may benefit patients who do not respond to lithium prophylaxis. The problem of treatment non-adherence may be dealt with through early identification of potential non-compliers and through the examination of the reasons why some patients discontinue lithium treatment against medical advice.

Identification of patients who respond to lithium prophylaxis

Various patient, illness and treatment variables which may predict good response to prophylactic treatment have been described by Carroll (1979) and Pétursson (1979). However, the relative contribution of many different demographic, clinical, genetic, biological and sociomedical variables to treatment outcome has been analysed only by Grof and associates who used multivariate statistics (Grof *et al.*, 1979, 1983). They showed that good response to long-term lithium treatment was related primarily to three clinical variables: (*a*) recurrent primary affective disease with a clearly episodic course, (*b*) intervals free of psychopathology and (*c*) a relatively low number of recent manic-depressive episodes or the absence of rapid cycling. Other variables also examined were either contained in the three clinical variables mentioned above or did not contribute to the variation in outcome. The predictive value of these three variables has been shown in studies by Grof *et al.* (1983) to be high; the outcome of prophylactic lithium treatment could be predicted correctly in 21 out of 24 patients.

The studies by Grof and associates have not yet been replicated by others. The examination of still other variables may add to the possibilities of predicting the response to prophylactic lithium treatment. In an on-going prospective study at the Psychiatric Hospital at Risskov in Denmark, special emphasis is placed on the identification of sociomedical predictors such as the patients' marital status, housing and occupation, etc.

Research methods which reliably identify predictors of treatment response may assist in creating multiaxial classifications which will give the most precise and comprehensive basis for decisions about long-term lithium treatment.

Alternative and combined prophylactic treatments

Drugs

Whether identified by the use of today's trial-and-error principle or tomorrow's use of sophisticated multiaxial diagnostic systems some patients inside the crude diagnostic framework of manic-depressive disorder will not respond to lithium and therefore need alternative or additional treatment. The same need will apply to those patients who, for various reasons, do not tolerate or accept lithium. Several psychotropic and non-psychotropic drugs have been tested. Some bipolar patients with predominantly manic episodes may benefit from long-term treatment with antipsychotic drugs (Ahlfors *et al.*, 1981), but bipolar patients should not be treated with antidepressants because this procedure is apt to precipitate manias. Unipolar patients may benefit from long-term treatment with antidepressants (Medical Research Council Drug Trials Subcommittee, 1981) but not from treatment with antipsychotics. Outside the group of psychotropic drugs, thyroid hormone and antiepileptics seem to be the most promising alternatives for some patients with manic-depressive disorder. Stancer & Persad (1982) showed that rapidly cycling manic-depressive patients benefited from levothyroxin treatment, an observation which is in accordance with observations from the 1920s of a beneficial effect of thyroid hormone given to patients with periodic catatonia

(Gjessing, 1983). The antiepileptic substance carbamazepine is the drug which has been most systematically examined as an alternative to lithium. In several open studies (Kisimoto *et al.*, 1983; Nolen, 1983) and in one controlled study (Okuma *et al.*, 1981) carbamazepine was shown to possess prophylactic efficacy in bipolar manic-depressive patients, probably being most effective in preventing manic episodes. Carbamazepine seems to be especially effective in patients with frequent episodes and in patients characterized as rapid cyclers (subgroups of patients which are least responsive to lithium prophylaxis). A number of patients have received carbamazepine treatment together with lithium for several years without adverse effects; one report (Chaudhry & Waters, 1983) does, however, warn against lithium and carbamazepine interaction as the authors observed one patient who developed severe neurotoxic symptoms during the combined treatment.

Psychotherapy

Various drugs may serve as alternatives or supplements to prophylactic lithium treatment. Psychotherapy is not an alternative to lithium prophylaxis but may serve as a very useful supplement. The aim of additional psychotherapy may be oriented towards greater insight; through prevention or amelioration of episodes, lithium treatment may render such therapy possible. The aim of psychotherapy may also be more modest, directed towards problems created by the illness and the treatment. Psychotherapy may serve to solve interpersonal problems which the patient encounters with spouse, family and colleagues and may support the treatment regimen through prevention of non-compliance. Jamison & Goodwin (1983) have given a thorough description of the possibilities offered by (supportive) psychotherapy to patients in prophylactic lithium treatment. They discuss issues such as the patients' experience of losses associated with lithium therapy, the patients' fear of recurrences, their denial of the illness, and their concerns about self development, family life and genetic consequences. The authors also discuss the important countertransference problems associated with psychotherapy of manic-depressive patients.

Compared with the number of studies carried out to examine the combined effect of psychotherapy and treatment with antipsychotic drugs in schizophrenia (Schooler, 1978) and with antidepressants in depressive patients (Weissman *et al.*, 1979), the number of studies dealing with the combined effect of psychotherapy and lithium treatment is small. Furthermore, these studies have considered different techniques; some deal with families (Keith, 1980), some with couples (Davenport *et al.*, 1977) and still others with groups (Volkmar *et al.*, 1980). None has examined the combination of individual psychotherapy and lithium treatment. Although fraught with methodological shortcomings, the studies offer many interesting clinical observations and altogether support the value of combining prophylactic lithium treatment with psychological intervention.

The prevention of non-compliance

As many as 20–30% of patients may discontinue prophylactic lithium treatment prematurely (van Putten & Jamison, 1980). The majority do so already during the first 6 months of treatment, long before a meaningful evaluation of the prophylactic efficacy of the treatment is possible. A few patients discontinue lithium in agreement with their doctors after renewed consideration of the diagnosis; the majority, however, discontinue lithium treatment against (or without) medical advice for a variety of reasons which have only been partly clarified. The reasons include somatic complaints as well as psychological stresses, often a mixture of both.

The somatic complaints refer to side effects which may develop during long-term lithium treatment. In a Danish study (Vestergaard, Amdisen & Schou, 1980) only 10% of 237 patients in long-term treatment did not suffer from somatic side effects, and 25% had more than three major complaints. Most troublesome and most often cited as reasons for discontinuing lithium treatment were weight gain, tremor, and polyuria/nycturia. The average serum lithium level was 0.83 mmol l^{-1}. In a more recent study in which lower serum lithium levels were applied (average 0.68 mmol l^{-1}) 40–50% of the patients did not complain of side effects (Vestergaard, 1983*b*).

Psychological factors which may lead to discontinuation of otherwise well indicated lithium prophylaxis have been studied by Jamison, Gerner & Goodwin (1979) and Jamison & Goodwin (1983). They included the following: the patients were bothered by the idea that moods were controlled by medication; they felt depressed; they were bothered by the idea of chronic illness, symbolized by the necessity of lithium treatment; and they missed the manic or hypomanic highs of bipolar illness.

Studies on patient attitudes towards the illness and towards lithium treatment may also reflect the reasons why some patients discontinue prophylactic lithium treatment prematurely. Jamison, Gerner & Hammen (1980) found that some patients felt the bipolar illness had made positive contributions to their lives through increased sexuality, productivity, creativity and sociability. Vestergaard & Amdisen (1983) found that of 140 patients given lithium treatment for 2–17 years, 25% perceived no other advantages than possibly the satisfaction of demands from family or doctor, and 70% of the patients considered various somatic and non-somatic complaints a main disadvantage of lithium treatment. Psychological and other non-somatic complaints related to work, training, patient status and the administration of lithium tablets were found, in the study by Vestergaard & Amdisen (1983), to be as frequent as somatic complaints.

Patient non-compliance may be prevented through identification of patients who are liable to discontinue treatment prematurely. In an on-going study at the Psychiatric Hospital at Risskov in Denmark, attempts are being made to identify demographic, clinical and sociomedical variables associated with non-compliance. If patients liable to non-compliant behaviour can be identified before prophylactic lithium treatment is started, special measures in treatment control may be implemented. Such measures may include frequent control, additional treatments, and attendance at a lithium clinic with specially skilled and experienced staff.

Conclusion

Long-term lithium prophylaxis is still the treatment of choice for the majority of patients with recurrent manic-depressive illness. Patients who do not respond fully to lithium and patients who do not tolerate or accept lithium may instead receive antipsychotic drugs (bipolar patients with predominantly manic episodes) or antidepressant drugs (unipolar patients). They may also be treated with antiepileptics, such as carbamazepine, given together with lithium or instead of lithium. Carbamazepine may be indicated for patients with frequent episodes and rapid cycles. In addition, patients may benefit from psychotherapy for solution of problems related to the illness and the treatment; psychotherapy may help patients accept the psychological problems inherent to long-term drug therapy. An optimum treatment regimen will help patients tolerate lithium. Most important is the prevention of side effects; this can be achieved through a maintenance regimen with serum lithium levels held at the lowest effective values. For the majority of manic-depressive patients in lithium prophylaxis, serum lithium levels between 0.5 and 0.8 mmol l^{-1} will be adequate.

References

Ahlfors, U. G., Baastrup, P. C., Dencker, S. J., Elgen, K., Lingjærde, O., Pedersen, V., Schou, M. & Aaskoven, O. (1981). Flupenthixol decanoate in recurrent manic-depressive illness: a comparison with lithium. *Acta Psychiatrica Scandinavica*, **64**, 226–37.

Carroll, B. J. (1979). Prediction of treatment outcome with lithium. *Archives of General Psychiatry*, **36**, 870–8.

Chaudhry, R. P. & Waters, R. G. H. (1983). Lithium and carbamazepine interaction: possible neurotoxicity. *Journal of Clinical Psychiatry*, **44**, 30–1.

Davenport, Y. B., Ebert, M. H., Adland, M. L. & Goodwin, F. K. (1977). Couples group therapy as an adjunct to lithium maintenance of the manic patient. *American Journal of Orthopsychiatry*, **47**, 495–502.

Gjessing, L. R. (1983). An essay on the syndrome of catatonia periodica. In *Neurobiology of Periodic Psychoses*, ed. N. Hatotani & J. Nomura, 15–45. Tokyo-New York: Igaku-Shoin.

Grof, P., Lane, J., Hux, M., Daigle, L., Grof, E. and Werstiuk, E. (1983). Predicting the response to long-term lithium treatment. Interim results of a prospective study. In *La Prédiction de la response au lithium*, ed. H. Dufour, D. Pringuey & T. Milech, pp. 165–70. Marseille.

Grof, P., Lane, J., MacCrimmon, D., Werstiuk, E., Blajchman, M., Daigle, L. & Varma, R. (1979). Clinical laboratory correlates of the response to long-term lithium treatment. In *Origin, Prevention and Treatment of Affective Disorders*, ed. M. Schou & E. Strömgren, pp. 28–40. London: Academic Press.

Jamison, K. R., Gerner, R. H. & Goodwin, F. K. (1979). Patient and physician attitudes towards lithium: relationship to compliance. *Archives of General Psychiatry*, **36**, 866–9.

Jamison, K. R., Gerner, R. H., Hammen, D. (1980). Clouds and silver linings: positive experiences associated with the primary affective disorders. *American Journal of Psychiatry*, **137**, 198–202.

Jamison, K. R. & Goodwin, F. K. (1983). Psychotherapeutic issues in bipolar illness. In *Psychiatry Update*, vol. 2. ed. L. Grinspoon, pp. 319–45. Washington DC: American Psychiatric Press, Inc.

Keith, D. V. (1980). Family therapy and lithium deficiency. *Journal of Marital and Family Therapy*, **6**, 49–53.

Kisimoto, A., Ogura, C., Hazama, H. & Inoque, K. (1983). Long-term prophylactic effects of carbamazepine in affective disorder. *British Journal of Psychiatry*, **143**, 327–31.

Medical Reserch Council Drug Trials Subcommittee (1981). Continuation therapy with lithium and amitriptyline in unipolar depressive illness: a controlled clinical trial. *Psychological Medicine*, **11**, 409–16.

Nolen, W. A. (1983). Carbamazepine, a possible adjunct or alternative to lithium in bipolar disorder. *Acta Psychiatrica Scandinavica*, **67**, 218–25.

Okuma, T., Inanaga, K., Otsuki, S., Sarai, K., Takahashi, R., Hazama, H., Mori, A. & Watanabe, S. (1981). A preliminary double-blind study on the efficacy of carbamazepine in prophylaxis of manic-depressive illness. *Psychopharmacology*, **73**, 95–6.

Pétursson, H. (1979). Prediction of lithium response. *Comprehensive Psychiatry*, **20**, 226–41.

Schooler, N. R. (1978). Antipsychotic drugs and psychological treatment in schizophrenia. In *Psychopharmacology: A Generation of Progress*, ed. M. A. Lipson, A. DiMascio & K. F. Killam. New York: Raven Press.

Schou, M. (1979*a*). Lithium prophylaxis: is the honeymoon over? *Australian and New Zealand Journal of Psychiatry*, **13**, 109–14.

Schou, M. (1979*b*). Lithium as a prophylactic agent in unipolar affective illness: comparison with cyclic antidepressants. *Archives of General Psychiatry*, **36**, 849–51.

Stancer, H. C. & Persad, E. (1982). Treatment of intractable rapid-cycling manic-depressive disorder with levothyroxine. *Archives of General Psychiatry*, **39**, 311–12.

van Putten, T. & Jamison, K. R. (1980). Rejection of lithium maintenance therapy by the patient. In *Handbook of Lithium Therapy*, ed. F. Neil Johnson. Lancaster: MTP Press.

Vestergaard, P. (1983*a*). Clinically important side effects of long-term lithium treatment: a review. *Acta Psychiatry Scandinavica*, **67**, Suppl. 305, 1–36.

Vestergaard, P. (1983*b*). Prophylactic lithium treatment with low serum levels. Paper presented at the VII World Congress of Psychiatry, Vienna, 1983.

Vestergaard, P. & Amdisen, A. (1983). Patient attitudes towards lithium. *Acta Psychiatrica Scandinavica*, **67**, 8–12.

Vestergaard, P., Amdisen, A. & Schou, M. (1980). Clinically significant side effects of lithium treatment. A survey of 237 patients in long-term treatment. *Acta Psychiatrica Scandinavica*, **62**, 193–200.

Volkmar, F. R., Bacon, S., Shakir, S. & Pfefferbaum, A. (1981). Group therapy in the management of manic-depressive illness. *American Journal of Psychotherapy*, **35**, 226–33.

Weissman, M. M., Prusoff, B. A., DiMascio, Neu, C., Goklaney, M. & Klerman, L. (1979). The efficacy of drugs and psychotherapy in the treatment of acute depression episodes. *American Journal of Psychiatry*, **136**, 555–8.

New perspectives in psychopharmacology

O. J. RAFAELSEN

From the breakthrough in psychopharmacology in the 1950s, the next 20 years were spent consolidating the bridgeheads both in theory and in practice. What is needed to-day is differentiation in the use of more specific drugs in more precisely defined groups of patients; it is my tenet that this next step will only be accomplished by 'operationalization' and integration of what is actually already in our hands. I shall use the monoamineoxidase inhibitors to illustrate the following points.

1. Operationalization and standardization of clinical assessment.
2. Application of more specific drugs.
3. Monitoring of the more relevant changes induced by treatment (*a*) biochemically, (*b*) pharmacologically and (*c*) clinically.

Why monoamineoxidase inhibitors? Because they were, in the early 1950s at the forefront of the first wave of new drugs and enthusiasm but, due to the lack of the tools and understanding I now hope for, they fell into ill-repute and were abandoned by most clinicians, even by whole countries.

Operationalization and standardization of clinical assessment

For nearly 40 years, clinicians have had the feeling that there were types of depressions responding better or only to monoamine oxidase (MAO)-inhibitors. But whenever it was tried to prove this tenet by comparisons in well-planned studies, the results were disappointing. The most notorious case was the British Medical Research Council study from 1965 where the MAO-inhibitor phenelzine was found to be inferior not only to electroconvulsive therapy (ECT) and to imipramine, but also to a placebo – the latter difference was, fortunately enough, not statistically significant (Shepherd, 1965). Ever since, many clinicians have argued that it was indeed the atypical depressive patients who were candidates for MAO-inhibitor (MAOI) treatment and that such patients rarely entered psychiatric hospitals and departments and that it therefore was not surprising that the results with hospitalized patients were rather disappointing (Quitkin *et al.*, 1981).

So what is atypical depression? Many will say that, compared to classical endogenous depression (melancholia), it is depressive states characterized by

1. phasic course less pronounced with long-lasting symptom-free periods;
2. no diurnal variation, but often with day-to-day variation;
3. mood change less marked, less total, less pitiful;
4. anxiety more prominent than in depression;
5. irritability instead of self-reproach;
6. demands and active appeal instead of excuses and passive appeal;
7. reactivity to personal contacts.

The results of Giller and his co-workers (1982) are along such lines. They compared Marplan® (= isocarboxazide) with placebo and found *trends* suggesting that the markedly improved group showed less depression, less anxiety, fewer sleep disturbances, less weight loss and fewer gastrointestinal complaints, but more helplessness and worthlessness. Others have also had to conclude that there were only weak differences in the profile between a tricyclic antidepressant like amitriptyline and a MAOI like phenelzine – amitriptyline producing greater improvement in depressive impairment of work and interests while phenelzine produces more improvement in anxiety ratings (Rowan *et al.*, 1981). Nies & Robinson (1981) compared the same two drugs and found no differences in total symptom severity or in patients with 'fears of recent onset'; they suggested, however, that phenelzine might be particularly efficacious in treating patients whose symptomatology included 'social fears'.

When treating neurotic patients with phenelzine or diazepam, Martin Roth and his group found no evidence of a difference in pattern of response between the two treatment groups and it was not possible to predict response to treatment from pretreatment variables (Mountjoy *et al.*, 1980).

A new approach was undertaken by Davidson and his group when making operational definitions of typical and atypical depression: 'We define typical depression as a state which is associated with loss of any of the following: appetite, weight or libido. Atypical depression is the converse, namely a gain in any of the above' (Davidson *et al.*, 1982). Their results, applying this very simple set of distinctions, were remarkable. The 'typical' depressions did not do significantly better on isocarboxazide than on placebo (although a uniform trend was noted which favoured the MAOI), whereas the 'atypical' depressions receiving isocarboxazide showed significantly greater improvement than those atypical cases receiving placebo on items of depression, anxiety, phobia, sensibility somatization, and obsession (Davidson *et al.*, 1981). This study, by its simple operationalizations of typical and atypical depression, invites replication studies to falsify or verify this interesting tenet.

Chemical Specificity

For many years it was not known that the MAO enzyme exists in two forms: (*a*) MAO type A (MAO-A; its preferred substrates include serotonin and noradrenaline) and (*b*) MAO type B (MAO-B; its preferred substrates include 'trace' amines such as phenylethylamine). Dopamine seems to be preferentially deaminated by MAO-B – at least in humans – whereas tyramine is a good substrate for both forms of the MAO enzyme.

Most of the MAOI are nonselective, i.e., they inhibit both MAO-A and MOA-B, but a few are selective. Clorgyline is a selective inhibitor of MAO-A, whereas pargyline and deprenaline (Deprenyl) are selective inhibitors of MAO-B. It was hoped that one or other type of selective MAO-inhibitors would have a more favourable ratio between wanted and unwanted effects, but these hopes have as yet not been substantiated.

It has been reported that clorgyline had stronger antidepressive effect than pargyline (Lipper *et al.*, 1979), but it has also been found that the enhancement of pressor sensitivity to tyramine, the most important adverse biological effect of MAO-inhibition, was stronger with clorgyline than with pargyline (Pickar *et al.*, 1981); in these studies both the wanted and the unwanted effects seemed to be more related to MAO-A than to MAO-B and thus chemical specificity did not immediately open up for a specific therapeutic advantage.

Monitoring of the relevant changes induced by treatment

The various reviews are immediately confronted with the crucial problem of how one can discuss efficacy without first defining the patient population? (Quitkin, Rifkin & Klein, 1979).

Suffice it to say that a majority of phenelzine-placebo studies showed positive effects in non-endogenous depression, whereas the results were modest or zero, compared with placebo in some important studies of endogenous depression (Greenblatt, Grosser & Wechsler, 1964; Shepherd, 1965; Raskin *et al.*, 1974).

Attempts have been made to explain some of the inherent problems pharmacodynamically and pharmacokinetically. Pharmacodynamics includes effective dosage and duration of treatment. Inhibition of at least 80% platelet-MAO led to clinical improvement in 68% of phenelzine treated patients, whereas only 44% of those with lower MAO-inhibition had a favourable response (Robinson *et al.*, 1978*a*). The same researchers found that with 60 mg of phenelzine, maximum platelet MAO-inhibition took more than 2 weeks to occur. (Robinson *et al.*, 1978*b*). We here see a possible explanation for the clinical observation that the full effect of MAO-inhibitor therapy takes 4–6 weeks.

It has been suggested that all MAO-inhibitor-treated patients should have a platelet-MAO-analysis after 3–4 weeks to ascertain whether sufficient MAO-inhibition has occurred, knowing the wide interindividual variation to drugs. This has at least not yet gained widespread acceptance, but it is evident that no patient has had an optimal chance to respond to this class of drugs if he has not had phenelzine at 60 mg per day, isocarboxazide at 30 mg per day, or other MAO-inhibitors at a similar dosage, for at least 4 weeks and preferably 6 weeks.

From a pharmacokinetic viewpoint, it is important that MAO-inhibitors partly are metabolized by acetylation. Individuals vary so considerably in their acetylation capacity that they can be divided into fast-acetylators and slow-acetylators. It was conceivable that this might influence the clinical response to MAO-inhibitor treatment, but investigations have failed to confirm this hypothesis.

Adrenaline has, in the last years, been recognized as a cerebral neurotransmitter in its own right. In two studies we have found very low cerebrospinal fluid (CSF)-adrenaline values in depression (whereas CSF-noradrenaline was not decreased). On clinical recovery CSF-adrenaline normalized (Christensen *et al.*, 1980; Gjerris *et al.*, 1981). In the rat we have recently been able to increase CSF-adrenaline by 250% over 6 weeks, whereas CSF-noradrenaline was only increased by 40% (A. Gjerris, *et al.*, 1984).

This indicates one of the crucial problems in research in general and psychopharmacology in particular. For many years research interests in depression and antidepressants centred around three amines: serotonin, noradrenaline and dopamine. Why these three neurotransmitters? Together they do not constitute more than about 1% of the estimated neurotransmitter substance of the brain! So what was their specific quality? Their distinction was that they could be visualized by fluorescent microscopy, and that glycine, acetylcholine, γ-aminobutyric acid and many others could *not*.

One of the newcomers to the family of *brain* neurotransmitters is good old adrenaline. It is only present in small amounts, but it is there. Da Prada and his group (1983) has found the change in brain adrenaline after a new reversible type-A-MAOI to be much more pronounced and longer lasting than that seen in brain noradrenaline. These results go hand in hand with our rat CSF-adrenaline changes after isocarboxazide, a mixed type, irreversible MAOI.

At present we have a clinical study in progress to see whether changes in human CSF-adrenaline 1 week after start of MAOI-therapy may predict clinical outcome, and whether its change is correlated to changes in operationalized clinical assessment as proposed by Davidson and his group. In this study we try to apply the principles I find important for new perspectives in psychopharmacology:

1. operationalization and standardization of clinical assessment;
2. application of more specific drugs;
3. monitoring of the more relevant changes induced by treatment (*a*) biochemically, (*b*) pharmacologically and (*c*) clinically.

Long-term therapy

Many clinicians have recognized that MAOI treatment was of long duration. Those patients responding to MAOI seemed to need it for many months, even many years. Very few studies have dealt with this problem which is one of the more difficult (but also more crucial) in psychopharmacology. In the Psychochemistry Out-Patient Clinic at the Rigshospitalet in Copenhagen, we have accumulated a number of patients, who have been receiving MAOI for up to 20 years (Larsen & Rafaelsen, 1980). Our study suffers from many of the classical problems being both open and retrospective; nevertheless the individual case records are very impressive. During the few weeks, 10 years ago, when one of the MAOIs was unavailable in Denmark, a couple of these patients relapsed.

Conclusion

Long-term studies in psychopharmacology are few and far between. With the attrition in patient numbers very few institutions can marshal the necessary patient material. Coordinated studies in Europe based on some of the principles mentioned in this presentation may bring us some of the answers we hope for.

Summary

There is a pronounced discrepancy between the number of studies of short-term treatments and of long-term treatments in psychiatry in general and in affective disorders in particular. The long-term studies have primarily dealt with lithium but, in fact, many more patients are in long-term therapy with cyclic antidepressants and, to a lesser extent, with MAO-inhibitors.

The new perspectives in *cyclic* antidepressants are (*a*) new drugs now available with less unwanted effects and less toxicity; (*b*) new drugs with different therapeutic profiles allowing a therapeutic sophistication; (*c*) for the same reason, and due to different mechanisms of action, these new drugs are also applicable as research tools in the elucidation of the biology of depressions.

The new perspectives in monoamine oxidase inhibitors (MAOI) are: (*a*) the increased use in long-term treatment; (*b*) the increased specificity of MAO-A and MAO-B inhibitors; (*c*) the demonstration of increased CSF-adrenaline after administration of MAOIs.

References

Christensen, N. J., Vestergaard, P., Sørensen, T. & Rafaelsen, O. J. (1980). Cerebrospinal fluid adrenaline and noradrenaline in depressed patients. *Acta Psychiatrica Scandinavica*, **61**, 178–82.

Da Prada, M., Kettler, R., Keller, H. H. & Haefely, W. E. (1983). Neurochemical effects *in vitro* and *in vivo* of the antidepressant Ro 11–1163, a specific and short-acting MAO-A inhibitor. *Modern Problems of Pharmacopsychiatry*, **19**, 231–45.

Davidson, J. R. T., Miller, R. D., Turnbull, D. C. & Sullivan, J. L. (1982). Atypical depression. *Archives of General Psychiatry*, **39**, 527–34.

Davidson, J., Weiss, J., Sullivan, J., Turnbull, C. & Linnoila, M. (1981). A placebo controlled evaluation of isocarboxazid in outpatients. In *Monoamine Oxidase Inhibitors*, eds M. B. H. Youdim & E. S. Paykel, pp. 115–24. Chichester: John Wiley & Sons Ltd.

Giller, E., Bialos, D., Riddle, M., Scholomskas, A. & Harkness, L. (1982). Monoamine oxidase inhibitor-responsive depression. *Psychiatry Research*, **6**, 41–8.

Gjerris, A., Barry, D. I., Christensen, M. J. & Rafaelsen, O. J. (1984). Brain and cerebrospinalfluid epinephrine in isocarboxacide and zimeldine treated rats. In *Catecholamines*, vol. 3, pp. 139–42, ed. E. Usdin, New York: in press.

Gjerris, A., Jensen, E., Christensen, N. J. & Rafaelsen, O. J. (1981). Adrenaline and noradrenaline in psychiatric disorders. In *Biological Psychiatry*, pp. 565–8. Amsterdam: Elsevier/North-Holland Biomedical Press.

Greenblatt, M., Grosser, G. H. & Wechsler, H. (1964). Differential response of hospitalized depressed patients in somatic therapy. *American Journal of Psychiatry*, **120**, 935–43.

Larsen, J. K. & Rafaelsen, O. J. (1980). Long-term treatment of depression with isocarboxazide. *Acta Psychiatrica Scandinavica*, **62**, 456–63.

Lipper, S., Murphy, D. L., Slater, S. & Buchsbaum, M. S. (1979). Comparative behavioral effects of clorgyline and pargyline in man: a preliminary report. *Psychopharmacology*, **62**, 123–8.

Mountjoy, C. Q., Marshall, E. F., Campbell, I. C., Garside, R. F. & Roth, M. (1980). Prediction of response to treatment with phenelzine in neurotic patients. *Progress in Neuro-Psychopharmacology*, **4**, 303–8.

Nies, A. & Robinson, D. S. (1981). Comparison of clinical effects of amitriptyline and phenelzine treatment. In *Monoamine Oxidase Inhibitors*, eds M. B. H. Youdim & E. S. Paykel, pp. 141–8. Chichester: John Wiley & Sons Ltd.

Pickar, D., Cohen, R. M., Jimerson, D. C., Lake, C. R. & Murphy, D. L. (1981). Tyramine infusions and selective MAO inhibitor treatment. II. Interrelationships among pressor sensitivity changes, platelet MAO inhibition and plasma MHPG reduction. *Psychopharmacology*, **74**, 8–12.

Quitkin, F. M., McGrath, P., Liebowitz, M. R., Steward, J. & Howard, A. (1981). Monoamine oxidase inhibitors in bipolar endogenous depressives. *Journal of Clinical Psychopharmacology*, **1**, 70–4.

Quitkin, F. M., Rifkin, A. & Klein, D. F. (1979). Monoamine oxidase inhibitors: a review of antidepressant effectiveness. *Archives of General Psychiatry*, **36**, 749–59.

Raskin, A., Schulterbrandt, J. G., Reatig, N., Crook, T. H. & Odle, D. (1974). Depression subtypes and response to phenelzine, diazepam, and a placebo. *Archives of General Psychiatry*, **30**, 66–75.

Robinson, D. S., Nies, A., Ravaris, C. L., Ives, J. O. & Bartlett, D. (1978*a*). Clinical pharmacology of phenelzine: MAO activity and clinical response. In *Psychopharmacology: A Generation of Progress*, eds M. Lipton, A. DiMascio & K. F. Killam, pp. 961–73. New York: Raven Press.

Robinson, D. S., Nies, A., Ravaris, C. L., Ives, J. O. & Bartlett, D. (1978*b*). Clinical pharmacology of phenelzine. *Archives of General Psychiatry*, **35**, 629–85.

Rowan, P. R., Paykel, E. S., Parker, R. R., Gatehouse, J. M. & Rao, B. M. (1981). Tricyclic anti-depressant and MAO-inhibitor: are there differential effects? In *Monoamine Oxidase Inhibitors*, eds M. B. H. Youdim & E. S. Paykel, pp. 125–39. Chichester: John Wiley & Sons Ltd.

Shepherd, M. (1965). Clinical trial of the treatment of depressive illness. *British Medical Journal*, **1**, 881–6.

Research implications of recent trends in the treatment of schizophrenia

L. CIOMPI

The purpose of this volume is, rather than looking for the right answers, to attempt more modestly to find some relevant *questions* for further research in the puzzling field of functional psychoses. Therefore, I want to start my chapter with a provocative statement about our ignorance concerning schizophrenia. In spite of 7–8 decades of continuous effort, we still do not know with sufficient precision what schizophrenia is, nor what are its limits, causes and best treatment. Worse, in the light of modern multifactorial, probabilistic, cybernetic and process-orientated scientific thinking, it becomes less and less certain that there exists such an illness as schizophrenia – or several schizophrenias – as a well-shaped disease entity with constant given causes, psychopathological picture and course. More likely, differing combinations of – certainly in part biological and in part psychosocial – factors might, in certain circumstances, converge (as is found in systems theory) towards more or less identical acute psychotic states which will then again split off into a wide variety of long-term evolutions which depend upon a great number of concomitant factors. Before focussing directly on my specific topic concerning therapy, I therefore feel the necessity to describe briefly certain important trends in the current understanding of schizophrenia and their slow but, as I believe, steady progress toward some useful overall hypotheses. Accordingly, I will discuss the following themes:

1. some general trends in the current understanding of schizophrenia: the 3-phase-model, the vulnerability-hypothesis, the information-processing hypothesis, and the distinction of the schizophrenic syndromes I and II;
2. two significant therapeutic trends: the prevention of acute relapses and the social rehabilitation of chronic schizophrenics; and
3. summary conclusions on some relevant questions for further research.

Some general trends in the current understanding of schizophrenia

As I have already discussed in detail on several other occasions (Ciompi, 1981, 1982, 1983), I think that the current knowledge of schizophrenia can best be summarized by the following *three-phase-model* (Fig. 1):

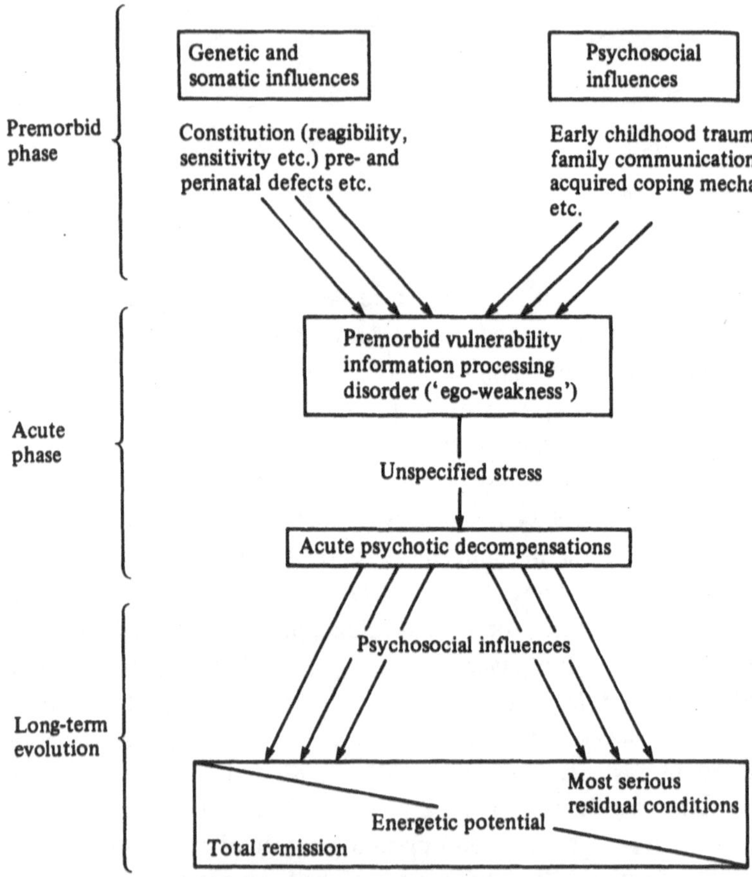

Fig. 1. Three-phase-model of schizophrenia.

In the *first*, *premorbid phase*, a variety of combinations of interacting biological and psychosocial factors (these may be genetically inborn, and/or pre or perinatally acquired, organic, e.g neurophysiological defects, unfavourable social and familial conditions, disturbed communication patterns, learning experiences, interpersonal relations, etc.) lead to a particular *premorbid vulnerability*. Its relative specificity is probably best described as an increased *difficulty in the adequate processing of complex information*. It must be emphasized that the concept of 'information' means here not only isolated experimental stimuli, easily measurable on a neurophysiological level, but also such highly complicated 'inputs' and 'messages' as the ones represented by long-lasting life-events and life-situations. As already described in my recent book on affectivity and logic (Ciompi, 1982), 'information' in this broad sense by no means includes only cognitive but also obligatorily *affective* elements.

It is probably through such complex affective-cognitive inputs mainly that the preexisting vulnerable equilibrium of the information-processing system can be critically overtaxed and destabilized in the *second phase*. Positive feed-back circles between biological and psychosocial influences in the sense of a 'runaway' (Bateson, 1979) or of 'fluctuations' (Prigogine & Stengers, 1981) may play a crucial role in the eventual *emergence of acute psychotic syndromes.*

What happens in the *third phase*, that is during the *long-term evolution* following the acute psychoses, seems again to depend on different combinations of a great number of factors, environmental and situational and probably also biological and constitutional. The recent long-term follow-up studies over several decades carried out by Bleuler (1972) and Huber, Gross & Schuettler (1979), to which we have contributed (Ciompi & Müller, 1976), with what are probably the longest existing follow-ups (289 cases with an average catamnesis of 36.9 years) have all shown that, in the long run, the evolutionary tendencies are more favourable, and particularly much more diverse than hitherto believed (Figs 2 and 3).

These interesting findings are now largely confirmed by several quite similar investigations, some of them still in progress, in the USA and in eastern countries (see Marinow, 1981; Sternberg, 1981; Harding *et al.*, 1982). Without going into the difficult discussion of the extent to which all these conditions were 'real schizophrenias' e.g. in the sense of the new Diagnostic and Statistical Manual of Mental Diseases of the American Medical Association (DSM III) – whilst I am convinced that at least in our material, the overwhelming majority was – it is obvious that for therapeutic and preventive purposes, this change in perspective has quite important implications. We know now that an initial schizophreniform psychosis, even if it lasts much more than 6 months, can completely disappear without leaving traces, or reappear once or several times, with or without combining itself with qualitatively quite different unproductive chronic syndromes of variable degree. Thus, instead of a steadily progressing fatality, the long-term evolutions appear now more like an open life process influenced and influencable by many factors, as well therapeutic ones.

It is not possible to present here details of all the evidence leading to such a modified view. This has been done extensively elsewhere (Ciompi,

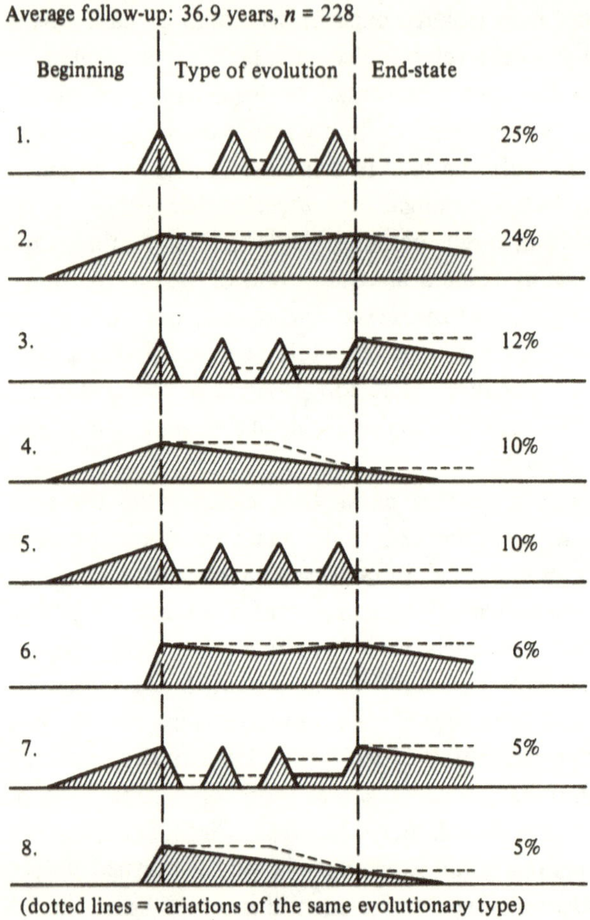

Fig. 2. Long-term evolution of schizophrenia (Ciompi & Müller, 1976).

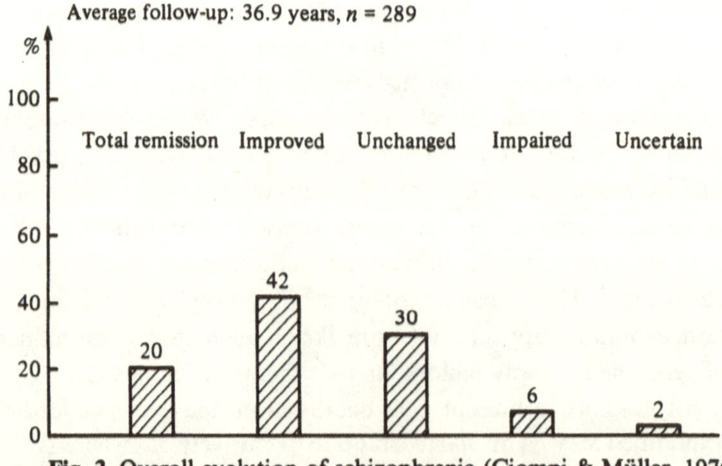

Fig. 3. Overall evolution of schizophrenia (Ciompi & Müller, 1976).

1980*a*, 1981, 1982). Let me just emphasize, before focussing on therapy, one more important development in our general understanding of schizophrenia: I mean the increasingly clear *distinction between the so-called productive or positive and the unproductive-negative syndromes* which currently are known under the designation of 'syndrome I' and 'syndrome II' introduced by Crow (1980, 1982), although they have been known under other names for a long time. Crow's interesting new hypothesis is however, that these so-different syndromes could have quite different and possibly even opposite causes, be these differences mainly biological (as Crow thinks) or psychosocial (as I formulated in a paper on chronic schizophrenia where the same hypothesis was enunciated independently; Ciompi, 1980*c*). This hypothesis, too, could lead to interesting new therapeutic approaches. Some should become apparent in discussion of our topic, that is to the research implications of recent therapeutic developments.

Two significant therapeutic trends: the prevention of acute relapses and the social rehabilitation of chronic patients

In my view, there are two main therapeutic fields where significant progress has been achieved during the last decade. On the one hand, the prevention of acute relapses during the initial stages of the illness (phase 2, Fig. 1) and, on the other, the social and vocational rehabilitation of long-term patients during the chronic stages (phase 3, Fig. 1). Both are essentially characterized, in close accordance with the previously mentioned general concepts, by a more and more sophisticated multifactorial approach.

Concerning the *prevention of acute relapses*, the clear evidence for the prophylactic efficiency of a long-lasting neuroleptic protection, following an acute episode (cf. e.g. Pietzker, 1978; May & Simpson, 1980), has now been completed by almost equally good evidence for additional favourable effects of certain psychosocial treatments. Authors like Hogarty *et al.* (1974), Goldstein *et al.* (1978), Falloon & Liberman (1983) and, most interestingly, Vaughn & Leff (1976*a*, *b*) and co-workers who continued the investigations initiated by Brown *et al.* (1962) in the 1960s have convincingly showed that the combination of drug treatment with systematic social support techniques, structured training of social skills, and especially with the diminution of the impact of hostility and emotional overinvolvement ('high expressed emotions') of close relatives reduces the relapse rate significantly. In their last and most differentiated approach, Leff *et al.* (1982) combined such techniques in a whole 'package' of interventions, including drug treatment, systematic education about schizophrenia for relatives, mixed high- and low-expressed-emotion (EE) multifamily groups, and family therapy. Several other authors, e.g. Anderson in the USA (1983) are currently working on similar lines.

The broadening of the therapeutic focus from the schizophrenic patient and his brain to significant parts of the surrounding social field provides (perhaps for the first time) some consistent, replicable and therapeutically applicable elements of insight into the complex interactions between exterior and interior, biological and psychosocial factors in schizophrenia. In line with the previously mentioned vulnerability and information-processing hypotheses, almost all the known therapeutic effects seem to converge, as I pointed out already in other reviews (Ciompi, 1982, 1983), at the conclusion that they *provide essentially a clarification and simplification of the informational input* in the formerly defined broad sense. In fact this is in my view the significant common denominator not only of the therapeutic effects obtained by transforming high-EE families into low-EE families, of the systematic education of the patient and his family on the nature of the illness, of the shaping of clearly structured treatment settings with easily understandable goals and proceedings, but of the positive effects of a reinforcement of familial hierarchies and interpersonal boundaries and of the minimization of contradictions and ambiguities noticed by dynamically orientated family therapists too. All these measures unify and order the surrounding communication field and simplify therefore the input of information it delivers. Even the action of neuroleptics can be interpreted as an improvement in information processing on different levels, e.g. through improved filter mechanisms and/or through the dampening of the affective components of information.

Consequently, this leads directly to the hypothesis that every kind of clarification and simplification of the incoming affective-cognitive stimuli, at least within a certain range or 'window' avoiding over- as well as understimulation (Wing, 1975), should result in a reduction of overt psychotic behavior and of relapse rates. Additional, and possibly quite important (but hitherto often neglected), aspects of the overall affective-cognitive input come thus in sight for further research, e.g. the *continuity of therapeutic programmes* and relationships over years instead of only months, the maintenance of such a continuity in spite of eventual changes from in-patient to out-patient or to halfway-care, the build-up of common, realistic, positive *expectations* in patients, families and therapists.

The *physical environment* of the patient too, e.g. the size and the architecture of hospital settings, the organization of admission wards, might be more important, in the light of the information-processing hypothesis, than generally admitted. If schizophrenia-prone people do really suffer from a critically reduced capacity to cope with complex information, then the usual big and agitated admission wards with their uninterrupted changes of nurses and of confused fellow-patients, their hardly understandable rites and procedures, their tension and oppression, the frequent changings from one ward and communication system to another, right at the beginning of the hospitalization should certainly all intensify the psychotic confusion.

Relevant questions for further research in this field might therefore be the testing, in addition to the already explored problems including drug-treatment, of the presumably positive therapeutic and preventive effects of clarity and continuity over sufficient periods of time versus confusion and discontinuity in:

- treatment programmes, procedures and goals;
- treatment settings and therapists involved;
- delivered information on the illness and its treatment;
- related internalized concepts and expectations in patients, relatives, nurses and therapists.

Several of these questions will be included in a research project which is currently in preparation in our institution. The *study of interactions of all these agents* under various conditions too, as already successfully initiated by several groups, obviously represents a central focus of future research.

One related, seemingly quite theoretical, question which has however many practical implications that we started to explore some time ago, concerns the *relations between the external sociofamilial structure and the corresponding internalized mental concepts.* According to Piaget and our own conceptualization (Ciompi, 1982) – which seems moreover, quite close to Janzarik's (1983) structural-dynamic views – the internalized 'programs' or 'affective-cognitive systems of reference' which determine the overt behaviour represent essentially a condensation of external actions and happenings, that is of the whole 'experience'. They can also be changed by new experiences (as for instance by clarified information and treatment procedures); a better understanding of these certainly circular relations would not only bridge the existing gap between a psycho- and a sociodynamic understanding but possibly also provide some new and useful tools for developing new behaviour-changing techniques.

A last very important question in this field concerns of course the favourable or unfavourable *effects of drugs in relation to the other mentioned factors.* Their dosage, necessary time of application, possible biological, psychological and social toxicity in the long run need more careful investigation. The time question is particularly far from being solved, as practically all the available studies on therapeutic and preventive measures cover only a few months or sometimes years, instead of the decades which are, in reality, required (our own long-term investigations have for instance shown that many formerly very severe schizophrenics remain absolutely symptom-free for decades without medication, while others suddenly relapse after very long delays with or without neuroleptic protection).

The second therapeutic area which seems to me particularly important is the *social and vocational rehabilitation of chronic schizophrenics*; it is my impression that publications (and, hence, also research interests) in this topic have somewhat diminished during the last years in favour of the focus on the combined treatment and prevention programmes I discussed before. It may be that several of the essentials of the rehabilitation techniques, of the organization of services, of possible results etc. have already been solved in the 1960s and early 1970s, through the pioneering investigations of such authors for instance as Wing (1963) and Bennett (1981) in England, Häfner & von Zerssen (1964) in Germany, Müller (1976; 1981) and to some extent ourselves (see below) in Switzerland. There is, however, no doubt that the practical development of rehabilitation services such as day- and night-hospitals, rehabilitation units, sheltered workshops, homes, apartments, crises-intervention units etc., as well as the refinement of techniques and concepts has steadily progressed in several places. Simultaneously, and in spite even of the economic recession, the number of long-stay patients in psychiatric hospitals continues to decrease. Related precisely to these developments, several new questions arise. I will briefly enumerate a few of them.

- The more the services are differentiated, the more *the problems of an optimal collaboration and continuity* over time between the different services involved become difficult to solve.
- In this field too, *the question of an optimal combination of different new approaches and techniques* – as, for instance, pharmacotherapy, training of social and vocational skills, family therapy or work with parental groups, individual or group psychotherapy and so on – is not yet adequately solved.
- The *relevant predictors and predominating factors influencing the success and failure* of rehabilitative efforts need further investigation.
- For evaluation research as well as for practical goal-setting, the problem of really *appropriate criteria for the definition of success and failure in social and vocational rehabilitation* is difficult to

solve (great individual variations in baselines and realistically reachable levels, multiplicity of involved aspects, value systems, environmental factors, etc.).

As an illustration of several of these problems I will refer to some of our own research in the field, published in a series of papers in German (Ciompi, Ague & Dauwalder, 1977, 1978; Ciompi, Dauwalder & Ague, 1979). We conceptualized social and vocational rehabilitation on two main axes: a *housing* and a *working axis* (Fig. 4).

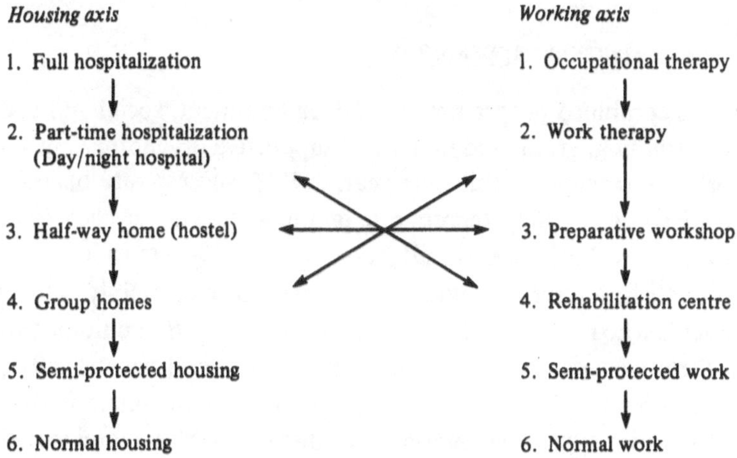

Fig. 4. Housing and working axis in rehabilitation.

These two axes can of course be flexibly combined – a patient will, for instance, stay for a long time in a sheltered home and move on the work axis, or stay in a rehabilitation unit and move on the housing axis – describe adequately a differentiated rehabilitation network. Goals as well as success or failure of rehabilitation can be clearly and even individually defined as levels to be reached on both axes, and appropriate programmes for reaching them can be designed on the basis of a systematic rating of the skills needed on each level through rating scales including – e.g. as in the scales we elaborated in our centre – the following items (Imfeld, 1977; Drezkowic-Parizek, 1980) for autonomous housing.

- eating habits;
- clothing;
- caring for a room or an apartment;
- utilizing public transport and communications;
- handling money;
- personal hygiene and health-care;
- coping with public services, officers and so on.

Similarly, for autonomous working, the following skills can be programmed:

- quality and quantity of work;
- regularity of presence, punctuality;
- working rhythm;
- concentration;
- behaviour with colleagues and superiors;
- working autonomy;
- personal appearance.

In a combined programme with drug treatment, social and vocational-skills training, group and individual supportive psychotherapy and family work, we reached, within one year, a 72% success rate on the housing axis (levels 4–6), 36% success rate on the work axis (levels 5–6) and 25% successes on both axes simultaneously. In a 10-year follow-up, E. Aebi (unpublished results) found among 107 chronic, mainly schizophrenic, patients who passed 6–18 months in our rehabilitation unit that about half of them were completely reintegrated socially and vocationally (53% in housing and 47% in work). The most interesting single finding of our investigations was that among the many variables examined, the (converging) initial expectations of the patient, of the nursing personnel and of the families were practically the best 1-year predictors of success or failure (Ciompi, Dauwalder & Ague, 1979). This surprising finding could recently be replicated even in a population of extremely chronified schizophrenic in-patients: 17% of them on the housing axis and 30% on the working axis (17% on both axes simultaneously) could still be rehabilitated within one year (Dauwalder *et al.*, 1984).

Such observations lead directly to the fundamental problem of *the nature of the chronic schizophrenic defect* and its possible reversibility or irreversibility as the essential limiting factor for all rehabilitative and therapeutic efforts. An intense discussion around this question, related to the concept of the so-called basic disorder, has again taken place in Germany (Huber, 1983; Janzarik, 1983; Mundt, 1983; Ciompi, 1980*c*); several summary statements on it, among them those of M. Bleuler (1983) and our own (Ciompi, 1983) which appeared recently in the *British Journal of Psychiatry* show a renewed interest in England too. The German authors see in these apparently irreversible 'basic disorders' the main expression of a permanent disorder in information processing; Süllwold (1977) proposes on this basis interesting training methods in order to minimize the effect of such defects. There are however still many unanswered questions. For instance, practically all long-term investigators report cases of late improvement, or even complete remission after many years and even decades of severe illness, involving apparently not only the so-called positive-productive but partly also the negative and unproductive symptomatology. This central question needs closer and more specific investigations than could be carried out in the follow-up studies mentioned.

Another important question which is still far from being solved, contrary to a widespread belief, concerns the *role played by genetic factors in the chronification of schizophrenia.* In most of the recent long-term investigations, heredity was *not* among the factors closely related to the long-term outcome. Bleuler (1972) found just some loose associations with the evolutionary forms; he quotes many authors with completely negative findings. In our own study (Ciompi & Müller, 1976, see also Ciompi, 1980*a*, *b*), there was no significant relationship at all. Huber *et al.* (1979) found paradoxically a statistical correlation between better evolutionary tendencies and higher hereditary loading. Several authors, among them Kety *et al.* (1976) reported however opposite results, that is a higher genetic loading in cases with more severe chronification. But these observations were generally based on smaller groups and much briefer periods of observation. The exact impact of genetics on the long-term course is therefore a question where specific research is surely needed.

On the other hand, there is now much evidence for the *influence of psychosocial factors on the long-term course*, such as the impact of the institutional milieu, of over- or understimulation (Wing & Brown, 1970) of life-events, of family dynamics, of the economic situation etc. (cf. Beck, 1978). In a comprehensive review which engendered quite a lot of discussion some years ago, I examined the arguments for and against the provocative thesis that an important part of the chronic schizophrenic defects and residual states could represent nothing other than a kind of a 'psychosocial artifact' (Ciompi, 1980*c*). Even if it was not possible to reach a final conclusion, the available data in favour of such a thesis seemed rather more plausible than the arguments of those against it. Anyhow, the question of the interactions between genetic or other biological factors on the one hand, and psychosocial variables on the other in long-term evolution is certainly just as fundamental for therapeutic purposes as the related one of reversibility or irreversibility of chronic states (not to speak of its interest for the general theory of schizophrenia).

There are, of course, many other questions of great weight. This includes research for other type of *drugs with better action on the negative-*

unproductive, chronic symptomatology than that of the ones which are currently available. It is closely linked to the question of the nature of the schizophrenic 'defect' and also to the mentioned hypothesis of a fundamental difference between the schizophrenic 'syndromes I and II'. The unsolved question of the *optimal time for application of drugs*, too, is of crucial importance in the long-term evolution (particularly with respect to possible, very severe side-effects such as tardive dyskinesia). As these problems lay however somewhat outside my specific field of work, I shall come to an end here and summarize, as a conclusion...not the answers but the most important *questions* which result from this brief overview.

Conclusions

First, I think that several additional elements of the possibly relevant informational input should be investigated under the overall hypothesis that a clarification and simplification of the incoming 'information' in a broad sense reduces the acute productive psychotic symptoms and the relapse rates. Among these elements to be studied special mention should be made of the continuity and the clarity of treatment programmes, the influence of the therapeutic setting, the constancy of well-structured therapeutic relationships over years (instead of months) and across several therapeutic institutions, the building up of realistically positive common expectations in patients, relatives and therapists.

Second, it seems crucial, in the prevention of acute relapses, to learn more about the individually most efficient, most economic and least damaging combination of therapeutic actions in a multifactorial biological and psychosocial approach, again taking into sufficient account the variable constellations and life-situations over a sufficient time. One particularly important aspect of this question is the optimal duration (in terms of long-term benefit) of different therapeutic measures including drug treatment, individual and/or family care, social and financial support etc.

Third, quite similar questions of continuity, clarity of programmes, optimal combination of the different elements of a multifactorial approach arise in relation to the specific problems of the social and vocational rehabilitation of chronic long-term patients.

Fourth, several fundamental questions related to chronic schizophrenia need urgently to be investigated, the most important being certainly the as yet unsolved problem of the nature and hence of the virtual reversibility or irreversibility of chronic conditions, especially of the so-called unproductive or negative symptoms. A closely related question concerns the role played respectively by genetic (or other possibly biological) and psychosocial factors in chronic schizophrenic evolutions.

Fifth, it is eminently desirable to intensify the search for drugs (or other therapeutic agents) with a better action on chronic unproductive schizophrenic conditions than those which are currently available.

References

Anderson, C. M. (1981). A psycho-educational model of family treatment for schizophrenia. In *Psychosocial Intervention in Schizophrenia*, eds H. Stiertin, L. C. Wynne, M. Wirsching, pp. 227–35. Berlin: Springer.

Bateson, G. (1979). *Mind and Nature. A necessary Unity*. New York: Dutton.

Beck, J. C. (1978). Social influences on the prognosis in schizophrenia. *Schizophrenia: Bulletin*, **4**, 86–101.

Bennett, D. H. (1981). Vocational aspects of rehabilitation. In *Rehabilitation of Patients with Schizophrenia and with Depressions*, eds J. K. Wing, P. Kielholz & W. M. Zinn. Bern-Stuttgart-Vienna: Huber.

Bleuler, M. (1972). *Die schizophrenen Geistesstörungen im Lichte langjähriger Kranken- und Familiengeschichten*. Stuttgart: Thieme.

Bleuler, M. (1983). Schizophrenic deterioration. *British Journal of Psychiatry*, **143**, 78–9.

Brown, G. W., Monck, E. M., Carstairs, G. M. & Wing, J. K. (1962). Influence of family life on the course of schizophrenic illness. *British Journal of Preventive and Social Medicine*, **16**, 55–68.

Ciompi, L. (1980*a*). The natural history of schizophrenia. *British Journal of Psychiatry*, **136**, 413–20.

Ciompi, L. (1980*b*). Catamnestic long-term study on the course of life and aging of schizophrenics. *Schizophrenia Bulletin*, **6**, 606–17.

Ciompi, L. (1980*c*). Ist die chronische Schizophrenie ein Artefakt? Argumente und Gegenargumente. *Fortschritte der Neurologie-Psychiatrie*, **48**, 237–48.

Ciompi, L. (1981). Wie können wir die Schizophrenen besser behandeln? Eine Synthese neuer Krankheits- und Therapiekonzepte. *Nervenarzt*, **52**, 506–15.

Ciompi, L. (1982). *Affektlogik. Über die Struktur der Psyche und ihre Entwicklung*. Ein Beitrag zur Schizophrenieforschung. Stuttgart: Klett-Cotta.

Ciompi, L. (1983). Schizophrenic deterioration. *British Journal of Psychiatry*, **143**, 79–80.

Ciompi, L. (1984). *Schizophrenie als Störung der Informationsverarbeitung. Eine Hypothese und ihre therapeutischen Konsequenzen*. In *Psychotherapie und Sozialtherapie der Schizophrenic*, ed. H. Stierlin, L. C. Wynne & M. Wirsching, pp. 59–72. Berlin: Springer Verlag.

Ciompi, L., Ague, C. & Dauwalder, J. P. (1977). Ein Forschungsprogramm zur Rehabilitation psychisch Kranker. I. Konzepte und methodologische Probleme. *Nervenarzt*, **48**, 12–18.

Ciompi, L., Ague, C. & Dauwalder, J. P. (1978). Ein Forschungsprogramm zur Rehabilitation psychisch Kranker. II. Querschnittsuntersuchung einer Population von chronischen Spitalpatienten. *Nervenarzt*, **49**, 232–8.

Ciompi, L., Dauwalder, J. P. & Ague, C. (1979). Ein Forschungsprogramm zur Rehabilitation psychisch Kranker. III. Längsschnittuntersuchungen zum Rehabilitationserfolg und zur Prognostik. *Nervenarzt*, **50**, 366–78.

Ciompi, L. & Müller, C. (1976). *Lebensweg und Alter der Schizophrenen. Eine katamnestische Langzeitstudie bis ins Senium*. Berlin, Heidelberg, New York: Springer.

Crow, T. J. (1980). Molecular pathology of schizophrenia: more than one disease process? *British Medical Journal*, **280**, 66–8.

Crow, T. J. (1982). Two syndromes of schizophrenia? *Trends in Neuroscience*, **5**, 351–4.

Dauwalder, H. P., Ciompi, L., Aebi, E. & Hubschmid, T. (1984). Ein Forschungsprogramm zur Rehabilitation psychisch Kranker. IV. Untersuchungen zur

Rolle von Zukunftserwartungen bei chronisch Schizophrenen. *Nervenarzt*, **55**, 257–64.

Drezkowicz-Parizek, J. (1980). *Konstruktion einer Schätzskala zum Sozialverhalten. Unveröffentlichte Lizentiatsarbeit.* University of Bern, Psychologisches Institut.

Falloon, R. H. & Liberman, R. P. (1983). Drug and psychosocial therapy in schizophrenia. *Schizophrenia Bulletin*, **9**, 543–54.

Goldstein, M., Rodwick, E. H., Evans, J., May, Ph. R. A. & Steinberg, M. R. (1978). Drug and family therapy in the aftercare of acute schizophrenics. *Archives of General Psychiatry*, **35**, 1169–77.

Häfner, H. & von Zerssen, D. (1964). Soziale Rehabilitation, ein integrierender Bestandteil psychischer Therapie. *Nervenarzt*, **35**, 242–7.

Harding, C. M., Brooks, G. W., Takamara, A. & Strauss, J. S. (1982). *What Happens to chronic psychiatric patients as they grow older? The Vermont Story.* NIMH-Conference on Schizophrenia, Paranoia and Schizophreniform Disorders in Later Life, Bethesda, 1–8 June. Guilford Press.

Hogarty, G. E., Goldberg, S. C., Schooler, N. R., Ulrich, R. F. & the Collaborative Study Group (1974). Drug and sociotherapy in the aftercare of schizophrenic patients. II. Two year relapse rate. *Archives of General Psychiatry*, **31**, 603–60.

Huber, G. (1983). Das Konzept substratnaher Basisstörungen und seine Bedeutung für Theorie und Therapie schizophrener Erkrankungen. *Nervenarzt*, **54**, 23–32.

Huber, G., Gross, G. & Schuettler, R. (1979). *Schizophrenie, eine Verlaufs- und sozialpsychiatrische Studie.* Berlin, Heidelberg, New York: Springer.

Janzarik, W. (1983). Basisstörungen. Eine Revision mit strukturdynamischen Mitteln. *Nervenarzt*, **54**, 122–30.

Imfeld, M.-Ch. (1977). *Berufliche Rehabilitatation ehemaliger psychiatrischer Patienten. Konstruktion einer Beobachtungsskala für Arbeitsverhalten.* University of Bern, Psychologisches Institut.

Kety, S. S., Rosenthal, D., Wender, H. & Schulsinger, F. (1976). Studies based on a total sample of adopted individuals and their relatives: why they were necessary, what they demonstrated and failed to demonstrate. *Schizophrenia Bulletin*, **2**, 413–28.

Leff, J., Kuipers, L., Berkowitz, R., Eberlein-Vries, R. & Sturgeon, D. (1982). A controlled trial of social intervention in the families of schizophrenic patients. *British Journal of Psychiatry*, **141**, 121–34.

Marinow, A. (1981). Über Verlauf, Ausgang und Prognose bei Schizophrenen. In *Schizophrenie. Stand und Entwicklungstendenzen der Forschung*, ed. G. Huber, (Hrsg.), p. 135–49. Stuttgart, New York: Schattauer.

May, P. R. A. & Simpson, G. M. (1980). Schizophrenia: evaluation of treatment methods. In *Comprehensive Textbook of Psychiatry* III, vol. 2, 3rd edn, eds H. I. Kaplan, A. M. Freedman & B. J. Sadock, pp. 1240–75. Baltimore, London: Williams & Wilkins.

Müller, C. (1976). Die Entwicklung vom Grossspital zur gemeindenahen Psychatrie. *Nervenarzt*, **47**, 295–9.

Müller, C. (1981). *Psychiatrische Institutionen. Ihre Möglichkeiten und Grenzen.* Berlin, Heidelberg, New York: Springer.

Mundt, Ch. (1983). Das residuale Apathiesyndrom der Schizophrenen. *Nervenarzt*, **54**, 131–8.

Pietzcker, A. (1978). Langzeitmedikation bei schizophrenen Kranken. *Nervenarzt*, **49**, 518–33.

Prigogine, I. & Stengers, I. (1981). *Dialog mit der Natur. Neue Wege naturwissenschaftlichen Denkens*, p. 202. München: Piper.

Sternberg, E. (1981). Verlaufsgesetzlichkeiten der Schizophrenie im Lichte von Langzeituntersuchungen bis ins Senium. In *Schizophrenie. Stand und Entwicklungstendenzen der Forschung*, ed. G. Huber (Hrsg.), p. 251–62. Stuttgart, New York: Schattauer.

Süllwold, L. (1977). *Symptome schizophrener Erkrankungen*. Berlin, Heidelberg, New York: Springer.

Vaughn, C. E. & Leff, J. P. (1976*a*). The influence of family and social factors on the course of psychiatric illness. *British Journal of Psychiatry*, **129**, 125–37.

Vaughn, C. E. & Leff, J. P. (1976*b*). The measurement of expressed emotion in the families of psychiatric patients. *British Journal of Social and Clinical Psychology*, **15**, 157–65.

Wing, J. K. (1963). Rehabilitation of psychiatric patients. *British Journal of Psychiatry*, **109**, 635–41.

Wing, J. K. (1975). Impairments in schizophrenia. In *Life History Research in Psychopathology*, vol. IV, eds R. Wirz, C. Winokur & M. Roff. Minneapolis: University of Minnesota Press.

Wing, J. K. & Brown, J. (1970). *Institutionalism and schizophrenia*. London: Cambridge University Press.

Long-term treatment of functional psychoses in childhood and adolescence

J. APPELBOOM-FONDU

Introduction

The diagnosis of 'functional psychosis' does not appear in recent infanto-juvenile literature. In our conception, we have deliberately decided to consider as a psychosis a psychic and behavioural mechanism elaborated against a primitive and existential anxiety. From this angle, every psychotic behaviour in childhood or adolescence (whatever its aetiology) can be considered as a functional psychosis. Infanto-juvenile psychosis can be considered from an analytical and intrapsychical, or a systemical and relational, or an organical and pharmacological point of view.

For psychoanalysts the crucial problem depends on the quality of the primitive relation between mother and child during his first year of life. Anxiety appears between 6 and 12 months of age; the resolution of this crucial phase in the personal development is essential. A lack of resolution may lead to severe behavioural troubles. The goal of therapy is to reach, through different media (like drawings, handling, games, body, words), those primitive problems.

From the systemic point of view, the patient is considered as the symptom of a dysfunctional family. The psychogenic family is centripetal; roles, limits are hidden and changing. Communications are chaotic or characterized by the double bind. Each tendency to attain a certain autonomy or a certain identity by one member of the family system provokes the elaboration of strategies to impede it and to preserve the homeostatic role of madness. Systemic psychotherapy consists of the clarification of the roles, limits and relations of every member of the family.

From the organic point of view, psychosis is considered as a genetically transmitted illness or as a congenital disease which stems from a defect in the metabolism of 3,4-dihydroxyphenylalanine (DOPA). During the last

5 years, research in this area in terms of the way in which it relates to children, has begun. In this context, treatment consists of the administration of drugs, associated (or not) with behavioural psychotherapy or pedagogic techniques. Literature concerning those approaches is relatively abundant although it is difficult to find comparative studies.

It is obvious that whatever the kind of psychotherapy, the result depends almost entirely on the relation between the therapist and his patient. Prognosis of the infanto-juvenile psychosis generally is not good: in the best conditions, psychosocial adaptation is relatively good but the fundamental problem remains intact.

Treatment of psychotic children

In a retrospective study, Rivière, Braconnier & Duche (1980) examined the role of precocity in diagnosis. From among 154 children who at the age of 3–7 years were being treated for psychosis, 39 were examined 15 years later. Each of them had been hospitalized in a psychiatric hospital and had had psychoanalytic psychotherapy. Two subgroups are described; the first was characterized by a symptomatology beginning before the age of 3 years; the second was characterized by a diagnosis after the age of 3 years. In the first group, evolution was better in terms of adaptability to every-day life, but they functioned in an oligophrenic manner. In the second, evolution was characterized by the appearance of critical episodes with delirium; they functioned in a schizoid manner. Some of them had a good evolution and, in those cases language ability has been shown before the age of 5 years and the intellectual potentialities were good.

Casadebaig & Exosteguy (1982) compared three types of treatment: ambulatory, evening and day. 90 children were investigated. It appears that ambulatory treatment has a positive effect on developmental problems or neurotic traits; a day structure has a positive effect on psychoses with sociofamilial interferences. Evening treatment has the best impact on neurotic children or on an old, functional psychotic population. The socio-economic status of these families is generally low. Evening treatment compensates for the defect of the family and helps school integration. Marcelli *et al.* (1981) insists on the importance of the hospitalization of these children. In his study, hospitalization of a psychotic child plays an important role in the family crisis, in the regression of the patient and his capacity for reconstruction. It also allows emergencies to be coped with.

A short stay in a pedopsychiatric hospital mobilizes affectivity: conflicts, reactions towards authority, problems of dependency and autonomy are more acute for the child and his family. During his stay in hospital, measures of placement are discussed. 30% are oriented to therapeutic homes, 8.5% to day-units, 5% are treated in an ambulatory unit, 4.5% are sent to new families. 52.5% stay in their own families. They are generally, neurotic patients. Concerning their mode of treatment: 49% take drugs, 21% receive psychotherapy, and 8% are treated with pedagogic or orthophonic measures.

The confrontation of these results with our own experience suggests that, as a first step, diagnosis is possible in an ambulatory regimen although behavioural observation sometimes implies day-hospitalization. The therapeutic phase requires brief hospitalization. Two factors appear to be complementary: the structural and the interactional. Hospital, family and child form a new relational system in which conflicts, separations and limits can be adjusted. A new homeostatic equilibrium for the family and the child can be found during this stay, relieving the child of the weight of his relational problems.

Later, a partial or total placement generally is necessary. The therapeutic approach would be an integration between institutional, individual and systemic cure. The institution brings on the confrontation between his phantasmatic and real life. Individual therapy reaches his underlying problems and gives him a personal territory with a privileged adult. Family therapy works with the interactions inside the system and so helps the integration of the child-symptom. Drug therapy improves the contact and thus helps the access to dialogue.

Treatment of psychotic adolescents

Normally, adolescence is a crisis period characterized by a revival of ancient problems, the contestation of myths and taboos previously accepted, and the anxious search for new reasons to live. Psychotic regression is sometimes an adaptive mechanism against this existential anxiety. 7% of psychiatric adolescents present acute psychotic decompensation. The signification of this symptom is different according to the context.

In some cases, a psychotic crisis is a positive experience that leads to maturation; in other cases, a psychotic crisis leads to psychiatric syndromes like schizophrenia or manic-depressive disorder. For De Negri & Moretti (1973), the therapeutic approach varies according to the premorbid personality. When it is abnormal, the evolution is slow and the treatment is mainly psychopedagogic and situational. When it is normal, a crisis is mostly treated by means of drugs. Evolution is variable. 20% of a population presenting a psychotic syndrome during adolescence become schizophrenic. Two specific ways have to be developed in the therapeutic approach to psychotic adolescents: crisis centres, community houses.

Crisis centres

These institutions are mainly indicated for young people living through a temporary social rupture and unable to overcome their difficulties with their common strategies. During such a stage, they are vulnerable and receptive to any kind of aid. For Caplan (1964), four phases are described:

- the impact of the stress,
- the disorganization,
- the mobilization of internal and external forces,
- the post-traumatic phase with the appearance of psychiatric syndromes.

Therapeutic intervention during a crisis period has different goals (Igodt, 1977): to absorb the confrontation with the stress, to maintain affectivity at a right level and to reach a change in the behaviour of the adolescent. Simultaneous action takes place in the family. The efficiency of this kind of approach is high. Adolescents accept these centres very easily because of the aid they offer and the opportunity for dialogue with emphatic adults who do not make a judgment upon them.

Community houses

In Denmark (Hoffmeyer, 1973) and France (Rault, 1981), 23% of psychotic adolescents are oriented to homes; 16% of them are oriented to community houses. These are generally located in the centre of the city and administered partially by adults and partially by adolescents. The adolescents who are sent to these communities are less disturbed from a functional point of view than those who are sent to crisis centres.

The goal of the placement is to create a new way of life for the adolescent, with new adults, new peers, new rules, new roles. Simultaneously, a therapeutic approach is used with the family and the therapeutic team to favour the future social reintegration of the patient in his family.

Conclusion

Therapeutic approach to psychotic children and adolescents is very complex because it implies different approaches which are not always compatible and therapeutic structures that vary with the severity of the symptomatology. Psychoanalytic, systemic, pedagogic, and drug approaches all seem to complete with each other so that no single technique can be considered superior to another.

At a structural level, it seems clear that mental health policies should put the emphasis on prevention. Early detection is of primordial importance.

Doctors, nurses and teachers need to be made more aware of early symptoms of psychosis. Therapeutic crisis centres have to be created in Europe with the aim of preventing relapses of psychiatric syndromes.

References

Caplan, G. (1964). *Principles of Preventative Psychiatry.* New York: Basic Books.

Casadebaig, F. & Exosteguy, N. (1982). Etude de l'indication thérapeutique 'unité de soins intensifs du soir' comparée aux indications thérapeutiques de 'cure ambulatoire' et 'hôpital de jour'. *La psychiatrie*, **25**, 423–8.

De Negri, M. & Moretti, G. (1973). Etude clinique des psychoses de l'adolescence. *Adolescentologie*, pp. 16–25. Milan: Carlo Erba.

Hoffmeyer, H. (1973). La psychiatrie de l'adolescence comme problème social. *Adolescentologie*, pp. 8–15. Milan: Carlo Erba.

Igodt, P. (1977). L'intervention en cas de crise. *Hospitalia*, **4**, 170–6.

Marcelli, D., Smarda, B. C., Carriere, N., Basquin, M., Duche, D. J. & Dugas, M. (1981). Hospitalisation en pédo-psychiatrie dans un hôpital général. *Neuropsychiatrie de l'Enfance*, **29**, 409–20.

Rault, A. (1981). Hospitalisation d'adolescents: des maisons dans la ville. *Neuropsychiatrie de l'Enfance*, **29**, 449–53.

Rauvet, M. & Ferrari, P. (1982). La sectorisation en psychiatrie infantojuvénile. *Neuropsychiatrie de l'Enfance*, **30**, 1–7.

Rivière, P., Braconnier, A. & Duche, D. J. (1980). Evolution des psychoses infantiles précoces. *Neuropsychiatrie de l'Enfance*, **28**, 117–31.

Seydoux, M. (1983). Les jeunes en crise et en rupture: réponses étrangères. *Neuropsychiatrie de l'Enfance*, **1**, 14–17.

Functional psychosis in old age

C. MÜLLER

While it is relatively easy to distinguish between functional and non-functional psychoses in adults, we find that matters become rather complex in old age, beginning let us say at the age of 65. There is almost always an overlapping of different factors, some of them specific to old age and others to the lifetime's experience of the individual. If we undertake to draw up a list of these factors, they would include the following.

The immediate environment

It is important in our pathogenetic hypotheses to note whether an aged person lives alone, in a family or in an institution. Social and affective isolation has been identified as one of the major factors in explaining psychic decompensation in the period of senescence.

The socioeconomic factor

It is a commonplace to assert that a person who has prepared for his retirement, who can carry out activities which interest him beyond the arbitrary limits of age, has a protective space around him against intolerable frustrations and against what Balier, has described in his theory of aging as 'the emptying of the positive content of narcissism, that is self esteem'.

Cerebral functioning

Physiological involution of the central nervous system appears, sooner or later, in old age. The variations are very great. We know centenarians with virtually intact intellectual capacities whereas, in other persons, reduction in the ability to adapt and learn, an impoverishment of imagination, and also a reduced capacity for storing engrams, are perceptible very early. Much has been said and written about the so-called involutive or psycho-organic element, in various functional psychoses of advanced years. While some authors attribute to this only a very secondary role and dispute the dogma of a 'defectology', others (on the basis of systematic investigations) demonstrate that a psycho-organic component may play a considerable role in triggering and maintaining functional psychoses in aged people.

Predispositions/personality traits

In our own studies, we have found that, despite certain accentuations, the character remains the same up to an advanced age and that even in the deepest demential states we can still recognize typical personality traits that have persisted throughout the life of the individual. These predispositions may therefore influence, if not the origin, at least the form and content of a functional psychosis. We have in mind, for example, the delusion of impoverishment, which establishes itself in a character marked by anxiety and obsession throughout the subject's lifetime.

Experience

What the individual has lived through and felt throughout his lifetime certainly has its importance in a functional psychosis in old age. This opens up the whole field of the evolution of psychotic patients who have undergone decompensation during adult life and continue to present psychotic symptomatology in advanced age. We shall return to this problem below.

Physical health

Polymorbidity is a familiar factor and nearly the most specific in psychogeriatrics. It must always be taken into account in our diagnostic considerations and therapeutic programmes, and also in our research. Thus, it is a matter of some importance in a delusional or hallucinating patient to recognize real disorders in the sensory domain, such as advanced deafness. In the same way, partial paralysis may naturally influence psychic equilibrium and have effects on maintaining the chronic state in psychosis.

To revert to the problem of distinguishing between functional and non-functional psychoses, we may go somewhat further and say that we can find functional elements in practically all psychopathological states in old age. Even advanced senile dementia, for example, may present symptoms, such as a confused condition, which we may characterize as functional.

To summarize, we may say that in principle every functional psychosis in old age has a multifactorial origin. This recognition renders it particularly difficult to make a schematic assessment and to isolate factors which could be the objects of systematic research.

Let us now consider some special aspects. Among the functional psychoses which appear for the first time in old age, without having been preceded by analogous conditions during adult life, we recognize above all involutional and senile depression, along with delirious states.

With regard to involutional depression, the question of classification remains open. Whereas some authors would like to identify it with either monopolar or bipolar endogenous depression, as listed in the World Health Organization (WHO) International Classification of Diseases (ICD), others would allow it a more independent status. Personally, I am inclined to consider this condition as having a special character, which distinguishes it from the endogenous depressions. The finding by Angst (1974) and his colleagues in Zurich that there is no fundamental difference between the so-called involutional depressions and the endogenous depressions of adult years with respect to hereditary factors is not, in my opinion, conclusive.

As for delusional states, the controversies also continue. While some authors tend to classify any delusional state which is not combined with a major and obvious psycho-organic syndrome as belonging to the domain of schizophrenia, others separate what one might call late schizophrenia from senile delusional states, continuing for example to use the term paraphrenia, a venerable word introduced into our vocabulary by Kraepelin (1896). However, as I attempted to demonstrate in the relevant chapter of my *Lexikon der Psychiatrie* (1973), this term now seems to me outdated, and we may note that it no longer appears in the ICD. It is in this context that we can verify our hypothesis that the origin of these delayed functional psychoses is multifactorial. What Janzarik (1981) masterfully described as 'Kontaktmangel Paranoïd' (paranoid evolution resulting from lack of contact), may be regarded as a model.

The boundary between a state of suspicion and mistrust in the aged person concerning those around him (who are felt to be hostile), and the emergence of true delusion is sometimes unclear. What is common to both the depressive states of senescence and delusional states is that therapeutic measures are especially difficult and that suicide is frequent.

Another aspect of functional psychosis in old age is that of the pharmacotoxic psychoses. Some authors tend to regard these types of acute exogenous reactions as functional psychoses *per se*. In a regular pattern, the patient first goes through a prodromal phase with discomfort, hypersensitivity and anxiety, followed by a phase marked by illusion and hallucination, difficulty in orientation and then enters into a confusional state which may reach the stage of coma. This destructurization in stages which Berner (1977) has described is fairly typical. Danielczyk (1979) systematically studied patients suffering from Parkinson's syndrome accompanied by vascular disorders. He found the same pattern. Among the drugs which triggered these exogenous reactions, he enumerated (in order of priority) antidepressants, neuroleptics, diuretics and digitalis.

Let us now turn to a problem which has been of concern to us in our service for many years: the aging of psychotic patients. We have re-examined several hundred schizophrenic and depressive patients 36.5 years on average after their first hospitalization; all of them were studied once they had already passed the limit age of 65 years. The results (Ciompi & Müller, 1976) are as follows. A modification of the symptomatology could be observed in some cases, but to a relatively minor extent. We never observed in the course of aging, for example, a case in which chronic schizophrenia evolved into a manic-depressive state, or vice versa. On the other hand, we did find that advanced age generally had a moderating effect on the preexisting psychoses, both with respect to the different forms of schizophrenia and endogenous depression, whether monopolar or bipolar. In the latter condition, we found that attacks diminish in intensity and that the symptomatology evolves more and more toward a syndrome of hypochondria and dysphoria.

In aging schizophrenics, we found a great variety of terminal states. Between the state of serious chronicity with major social handicap and that of a complete cure leaving no residue of the preceding psychosis, there is a wide range of possibilities. Differences between the subgroups of schizophrenia become blurred and, in old age, it is virtually impossible to recognize the difference between patients who started out with paranoid, hebephrenic or catatonic schizophrenia. This modification of schizophrenia in old age opens up interesting perspectives on various aetiopathogenetic hypotheses and it seems to us that no one has yet drawn all the possible conclusions on this subject. Simplifying matters a little, I might suggest for example that psychotic regression has given way to a more physiological regression in the service of the Self, to use the terminology of Kris (1967). We might also speak of adaptive regression or even of physiological regression.

Thus, at the end of his life, the chronic psychotic might be reverting, in a sense, to the neurotic equilibrium which preceded the psychotic decompensation and we could refer to neo-neuroticization. Such neuroticization might have a painless, egosyntonic character, and we could thus qualify it as an adaptive old age neurosis. In pursuing this line of thought

I am following the reflections of Andreoli & Quartier (1976) who, on the basis of a psychoanalytic concept, spoke of a general change in the flow of investments. In old age, external reality is progressively disinvested in favor of hyperinvestment in the self or in the past. While this movement of withdrawal into the self in a non-psychotic subject will engender a dangerous process (since the image he finds in his mirror will be disappointing), this new regression in an aged psychotic will be functional, since its purpose is the regressive diversion of psychic energy from relation to the object to place it at the disposal of the troubled Self.

Let us conclude then with the perspectives for research. There have been numerous epidemiological studies of the incidence of functional psychosis in old age. The English school, in particular, Bergmann (1960), Post (1962), Roth & Morrisey (1962) and others, has enriched our knowledge of the psychopathology in old age. In Germany, I would refer to the work of Cooper & Kunze (1979) which studied the frequency of psychic disorders in old age in relation to various social parameters. I do not believe that subsequent research in this field will bring us much in the way of surprises. I see the future of research in the field of functional psychoses in old age developing along two lines.

First, we should have a better understanding of the neurophysiological and neurochemical origins of the increased vulnerability of the aging brain. This vulnerability is manifest to the doctor, for example, by the fact that the old patient on the average needs only one-third of the dosage of psychotropic drugs given to a young adult. This line of research will obviously lead us to further study of the aging nerve cell.

Second, we should explore the field of psychological influences. In this domain, I have in mind especially the study of cases in detail, i.e. through lifespan studies. Here however we encounter a major methodological difficulty: prospective studies demonstrate that neither an individual researcher nor even a group of researchers can expect to have time enough to study the evolution of an adult individual up to old age; on the other hand, catamnestic studies can concern themselves only with the survivors whom they are able to follow (necessarily a selected population).

In a Latin verse, the old man tells us 'sum quod eris quod es ante fui' (I am what you will be, and what you are, I was). This is a kind of triumphalist position which should induce reflection upon the limits of our research possibilities. However, the human mind is marked by curiosity and it would be wrong to take refuge in any sort of resignation. Whether we like it or not, the increasing number of aged people, and the pathology they present, will oblige us to continue our efforts.

References

Andreoli, A. & Quartier, F. (1976). Repli et 'régression nevrotique' chez le vieillard. *Information psychiatrique*, **52**, 1155–65.

Angst, J. (ed.) (1974). *Classification and Prediction of Outcome of Depression*. Symposium Schloss Reinhartshausen/Rhein, Sept. 23–26 1973. Stuttgart: Schattauer.

Balier, C. Hygiène mentale du troisième âge. *Encyclopédie médico-chirurgicale. Psychiatrie*, **37960 G 10**, 1–6.

Bergmann, B. (1960). Über phantastische paranoisch-halluzinatorische Krankheitsbilder der höheren Lebensalters. *Schweizerischer Archiv für Neurologie, Neurochirurgie und Psychiatrie*, **86**, 192–207.

Berner, P. (1977). Körperlich begründbare Störungen. In *Psychiatrische Systematik*, unter Mitarbeit von K. Kryspin-Exner. 251. Bern: Huber.

Ciompi, L. & Müller, C. (1976). *Lebensweg und Alter der Schizophrenen*. Eine katamnestische Langzeitstudie bis ins Senium. Berlin: Springer.

Cooper, B. & Kunze, H. (1979). Sozialpsychiatrie. In *Die Psychologie des 20 Jahrhundert*, pp. 224–55. Zürich: Kindler.

Danielczyk, W. (1979). Akute pharmakotoxische Psychosen bei chronischen zerebralen Erkrankungen. *Wiener medizinische Wochenschrift*, **129**, suppl. 55, 3–15.

Janzarik, W. (1981). Situation, Struktur, Reaktion und Psychose. *Nervenarzt*, **52**, 396–400.

Kraepelin, E. (1896). *Lehrbuch der Psychiatrie*. Leipzig: Barth.

Kris, E. (1967). *Richerche Psicoanalitiche Sull'arte*. Torino: Einandi.

Müller, C. (1973). *Lexikon der Psychiatrie*. Berlin: Springer.

Post, F. (1962). *The Significance of Affective Symptoms in Old Age*. A follow-up study of one hundred patients. London: Oxford University Press.

Roth, M. & Morrisey, J. D. (1962). Problems in the diagnosis and classification of mental disorder in old age; with a study of material. *Journal of Mental Science*, **98**, 66–80.

Chronicity and hospitalization: can the vicious circles be broken?

A Finnish perspective on the need for experimental activities and follow-up studies in the integrated rehabilitation system of schizophrenic clients

E. E. ANTTINEN

An overview of mental health services in Finland

Up until the end of the 1960s, emphasis in the development of the Finnish mental health service system was rather heavily on hospital care. The number of psychiatric beds per 1000 inhabitants at the beginning of the 1980s was still 4.1. The development of out-patient care got under way during the 1960s and, at present, we have a relatively comprehensive network of mental health centres. Regional shortcomings still exist, however, and we still suffer from a lack of alternative forms of rehabilitation. The most serious difficulties are linked to the shortage of psychiatrists but also to shortages of specialized graduate nurses both in hospitals and in out-patient care.

Preventive mental health work, psychiatric care and rehabilitation has been organized in Finland by dividing the country into mental health care districts. The federations of communes responsible for providing the services in each district maintain (by government financial support) the hospitals, mental health centres and other services needed for out-patient care and rehabilitation. The provision of services is based on the Mental Health Act passed in 1952 and amended in 1978 which favours out-patient care and rehabilitation. Another Act, the 1972 Primary Health Care Act stipulates that the health centre network, led by general practitioners, should take the first line of responsibility in all health care and so support special services, including those concerned with psychiatric care.

The insufficient resources of out-patient care, the extensiveness of and consequent long distances within the mental health care districts, the fact that psychiatric care has earlier been concentrated in hospitals and that the ideology of sociotherapeutic care is rather recent in Finland, together with the public attitude, all underlie the problems of hospitalization in our country.

The following is an introduction to the situation in one mental health care district, especially in the light of the problems involved in rehabilitation of schizophrenics.

Research as an indicator of the need for development

The mental health district of North Häme covers an area of 8600 km² and some 321 000 inhabitants. There are a total of 1468 beds in the four psychiatric hospitals of the district, i.e. 4.5 beds per 1000 inhabitants. Out-patient visits to our mental health centres and psychiatric out-patient clinic total some 30 000 per year, i.e. 90 visits per 1000 inhabitants. These are 1982 figures.

We have carried out surveys of the rehabilitation potential and social circumstances of all hospital patients in 1965, 1967, 1973 and 1979. The one-day figures in the years mentioned ranged from 1460 to 1516 patients, the diagnosis of 50–60% of them being schizophrenia or suffering from paranoid psychosis. According to these one-day surveys, the absolute number of schizophrenic patients in our care units has during these 14 years varied from 773 to 827.

Among these schizophrenic patients, the main problems seemed to be loneliness, lack of practical possibilities (housing and work) of leading a normal life outside hospital, and insufficient social skills and emotional capacity. These features, bound up with chronicity and hospitalization, can be illustrated by the following figures. In the 1960s, the last period of hospitalization of almost 80% of schizophrenic patients was 2 years or more, in 1979 the figure was still 68%. The corresponding figures for those hospitalized five years or more were 66% and 54%. Of the patients in treatment during the 1960s 11% were married, in 1979 only 4.3% of schizophrenic patients had a spouse. Less than 30% of them could rely on support from relatives. For most of them, skills for work or job opportunities and prospects for finding housing were poor. Where hospitalization had continued for more than 2 years, bridges back to society began to weaken rapidly.

The above goes to show that high numbers of hospital beds in our district has also kept a great number of our schizophrenic patients in hospital: chronicity and hospitalization have been entangled in a vicious circle. But since the beginning of the 1970s this has not, at least to the same extent as earlier, been the cause among new schizophrenics entering hospital. Our 5-year follow-up study of patient groups suggests that their average period of hospitalization is relatively short, with only 18% using hospital care for longer periods. About half of the latter are most likely 'new long-stay' patients with a great potential for hospitalization.

Experimentation activities

Our search for alternatives to hospital care and rehabilitation was started in 1964. The principal objective of our experiments was to influence the factors that created the vicious circle of hospitalization and chronicity. There were two forms of activity that, to us, seemed most successful: (*a*) treatment and rehabilitation based on home visits, at first made quite frequently, and in which the family was taken as the unit of care, and (*b*) rehabilitation homes where those undergoing treatment formed small sociotherapeutic communities. Treatment and rehabilitation were both supervised by trained psychiatric nurses with flexible and close support and guidance by a psychiatrist.

The home care experiment

The study material in the home care experiment (Anttinen, Eloranta & Stenij, 1971) comprised 100 schizophrenics (and their families) successively discharged from hospital and living at home. Our reference group consisted of 169 schizophrenics in conventional out-patient care. The experiment lasted 2 years. The results were most promising:

- By creating a new extramural step of care between the hospital and the mental health centre, the possibilities of individual and family treatment were significantly improved.
- A statistically significant reduction in the need for hospital care was achieved in comparison with the reference group.
- The patients' ability to manage in sheltered work and to carry out various housework tasks improved considerably.
- In most cases, it was possible to influence the patients' psychic condition favourably.
- Repeated home visits and, later on, patients' visits to the out patient clinic allowed simultaneous guidance and treatment of both the patient and his family or other key persons. This integrated the patient more tightly to his small community in which he lived and at the same time eased the lives of several people; this resulted in a more therapeutic atmosphere at home.

However, there were 17 persons without family in the home care group. It was also found that some others had difficulties in personal relationships that in the long run overburdened the entire family community; further, problems arose where this severe illness in a family with children necessitated inconvenient arrangements. In all, it seemed that for some 30% of the home care patients the best solution would have been to be able to live in a rehabilitation home or hostel and to go out for day care or to sheltered work. At that time, however, such arrangements were not possible in our district.

Sociotherapy in small community
Our experiments extended in 1966 to a new alternative form of rehabilitation when the first sociotherapeutic hostel was established in the mental health district. Six schizophrenic women were admitted from the hospital to the hostel. All of these women had suffered from their illness for a long time; their last period of hospitalization had lasted 10–28 years. They were single, lonely women who had lost all their contacts outside the hospital.

After 2.5 years of an active, supportive yet independence-motivating group process led by the home care nurse and utilizing sociotherapeutic methods, all of the patients were able to lead an independent life outside the hostel. Having been at first withdrawn, passive, uncertain and emotionally difficult to approach, they gradually opened up. Five years later, one of them had died of a somatic disease, one had had to resort to brief periods of hospitalization, and four had managed well. They still showed symptoms of schizophrenia, but socially they were positively active and successful: they had become independent and responsible members of society.

Development and experimentation of the integrated rehabilitation system

Both the home care study and the sociotherapeutic rehabilitation experiment provided some practical starting-points for the development of the rehabilitation system for long-term schizophrenic hospital patients.

1. They must be guided away from the institution and from loneliness to a functioning, small, interacting network.
2. Every schizophrenic, including those with chronic and difficult syndromes, must be approached as a person and on equal terms; his self-esteem is to be strengthened, and he must be allowed to experience himself as a fellow human being.
3. With few exceptions, people who have suffered from long-term schizophrenia can (although often only very slowly) learn important activities and technical skills in sheltered circumstances. The illness itself, the attitudes in the patient's environment and evolving vicious circles do not allow this in unsheltered circumstances. The major obstacles are emotional and social difficulties.
4. The above constitutes a challenge to rehabilitation: it must, in all cases, combine psychotherapeutic and sociotherapeutic means in

teaching functional skills. Opportunities for rehabilitation must be offered in situations of everyday life, within the small interacting community, at work and in leisure activities.

These very ideas that I have discussed above have, of course been introduced in both earlier and more recent literature (e.g. Brown *et al.*, 1966; Jones, 1968; Edelson, 1970; Bleuler, 1972; Ciompi & Müller, 1976; Jones, 1978; Huber, Gross & Schüttler, 1979; Mosher & Keith, 1979; Ciompi, 1981; Wykes & Wing, 1982). It was these ideas that encouraged us to attempt to develop a comprehensive and integrated rehabilitation system for long-term schizophrenic patients. Also, these experiences paved the way for the adoption of the therapeutic community ideology as the most important instrument in rehabilitation work.

Inasmuch as legislation in 1970 did not enable such forms of activity as we felt necessary to be established within the public service system, we launched our programme under a private association. The association (Sopimusvuori Association) was established in May 1970 and has received communal subsidies from the outset. During its first year, it established a 21-place rehabilitation home and a partly supported hostel; over the past 12 years, it has continuously expanded and developed its activities.

At present, the association has 245 rehabilitation places. Activities are centred around the rehabilitation homes ($n = 6$, 69 places), small homes ($n = 6$, 28 places), supported lodgings or residences ($n = 19$, 34 places), the day care home ($n = 1$, 42 clients), the workshop ($n = 1$, 60 clients) and one so-called preventive rehabilitation home for special purposes (12 clients). The annual growth in the number of places (Table 1) has followed the needs of both the hospitals and the population in the mental health district in a flexible manner. The rehabilitation units form a progressive, graded system (Fig. 1) in which the client can, as rehabilitation advances, move on to the next step according to his abilities. Our objective has been to avoid radical jumps between these steps and to make the system as smooth, flexible and as non-bureaucratic as possible. It must encourage progress and it must allow setbacks. We have aimed at creating therapeutic communities where the clients and the staff work together on equal terms and without hierarchical arrangements. Rehabilitation programmes are individual and naturally, they are, drawn up together with the client.

Of the running expenses arising from the 245 rehabilitation places, 45% are covered by the clients, 43% by municipal subsidies and 12% by income from the workshop. The total cost per client day in 1982 was 40 FIM (USD8).

The total number of staff is 28, half of whom are specially trained

Table 1. *The trend in rehabilitation places of Sopimusvuori in 1970–1982*

	1970	1971	1972	1973	1974	1975	1976	1977	1978	1979	1980	1981	1982
Rehabilitation homes	20	21	37	41	47	67	69	69	68	67	69	63	69
Small homes						5	9	9	15	20	20	24	28
Supported hostels	6	19	34	34	38	45	33	29	23	11	11	4	—
Supported lodging or residences								4	12	18	18	27	34
Day care home (homes)		26	57	57	55	61	35	35	40	32	30	30	42
Workshop			20	20	30	40	60	60	60	60	60	60	60
Pirtti (preventive rehabilitation) home)							12	12	12	12	12	12	12
Total	26	66	148	156	170	218	218	218	230	220	220	220	245

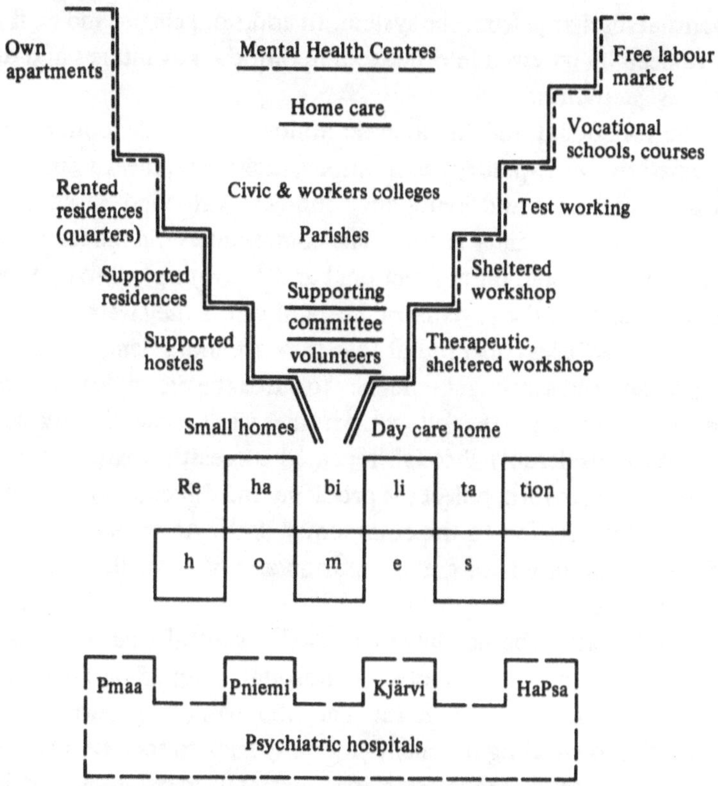

Fig. 1. Rehabilitation steps in North Häme mental health district for long term patients. Solid line, steps owned by Sopimusvuori Association; dotted line, clients supported by Sopimusvuori Association; dashed line, owned by mental health district.

psychiatric nurses. All staff members have also actively participated in complementary education. Occupational guidance is arranged on a regular basis. Moreover, a voluntary friendship society (friend service) supports the association's clients and activities.

Observations and research results

From 1972 onwards, the experimental activities have been closely followed by studies partly financed by the Academy of Finland and the National Board of Health (Ojanen & Saukkonen, 1975; Ojanen, 1978; Ojanen, 1980; Anttinen & Jokinen, 1982). The aim of this research work has been to gather experience for the further development of these activities. Special attention has been paid to the development of the atmosphere in the communities and to how they have met the 'criteria' of a therapeutic community. Another focus of study has been the change in the clients' social skills and their path through the various levels of and eventual discharge from the system. In addition, clients and staff members have been interviewed in order to pinpoint the advantages and difficulties of these activities.

The functional and therapeutic atmosphere of the communities were assessed by participatory observations, interviews, measurements (perception of treatment and living environment; a method based on work by R. H. Moos) and diary entries. The communities did indeed prove clearly more interactional, more functional and activating, more open and more democratic than the psychiatric hospital wards they were compared with. It was nevertheless also found that they are more demanding and in this respect showed a stronger tendency towards the principle of normality. An important finding in the follow-up studies was the fact that the community matures considerably through repeated successful treatment of common crises, which, in turn, reflect the problems and difficulties of the community members in relation to the community itself. As we see it, the maturing of the community is of great importance in view of the rehabilitation of its members.

Rehabilitation homes have assumed a central role in the attempt to break the vicious circle involved in hospitalization. Small homes, lodgings or residences, day care home and the workshop form the steps of rehabilitation leading the client gradually back to society. These levels can also sometimes be used as first steps in extramural treatment for chronically ill patients showing lesser symptoms when the patient cannot return directly to his occupation or home.

Next I shall discuss the results we obtained in following up the 201 rehabilitation home clients who first entered our integrated rehabilitation system. They represent the most hospitalized group of our clients since we started in 1970. At that time, 52% had spent more than 10 years and 65% more than 5 years in hospital. The former group comprised several patients who had a 30–40 year uninterrupted period of hospitalization behind them; the average year of birth in this group was around 1933. The follow-up studies among these 201 clients up until 1979 revealed that: 60% of them had gradually been able to move on to live in a supported lodging or residence, in a rented or self-owned flat, or together with their families. Follow-up studies have indicated that they generally have managed well. Only 9% of this group studied during the follow-up years had had to resort to temporary hospital care and only 9% – due to their worsened condition – had had to return to the rehabilitation home. For about 20% of the entire group the rehabilitation home is the highest level of rehabilitation ever needed. Finally, rehabilitation among the remaining 20% of the rehabilitation clients must be seen to have failed and that they have had to return to hospital, most likely permanently.

In all, over 500 clients have to date been transferred from hospitals to our rehabilitation homes. The results are, on average, more or less equally good: in 1982, for instance, 39 clients left our rehabilitation homes, of whom 3 moved to small homes or supported hostels, 9 went to a supported lodging or residence, 2 went to live with his/her parents and 16 moved to rented residences or apartments of their own. Nine of the clients returned to hospital.

In keeping with concepts advanced by others (Ciompi & Müller, 1976; Wing, 1976; Huber, Gross & Schüttler, 1979), these observations also showed that rehabilitation of a long-term hospital patient is often a slow process. Nonetheless, progress almost always does start at some stage, even if it might take 1–2 years before any signs become visible. According to the follow-up studies, our rehabilitation system is best able to help middle-aged and elderly female patients, while it offers the least support for young, single men. On the basis of these findings we agree with the points already raised by Bleuler (1972) and with those claiming that higher age correlates positively with the relief of psychotic symptoms, as Ciompi & Müller have pointed out. We would further want to underline that the rehabilitation potential of most long-term schizophrenics increases as they approach middle age – and that this is where rehabilitation has its second opportunity. The early, acute phase of the illness is definitely its first opportunity.

The overall quality of life and functional capacity of the clients who gradually move on from therapeutic communities in rehabilitation homes to lead an independent life in society are better than those among the control group patients discharged from hospital and living at home. The former are more independent and more active; also, overall death rates and suicide figures are slightly smaller among the former than among the latter group.

The communities of the rehabilitation homes, day care homes and the workshop and hostels are, as they stand today, a result of relatively long development processes that have, to some extent, differed from each other. Physicians have not participated directly in the communities' activities, and the number of care personnel in the communities has been kept at a minimum. The latter have mainly offered identificatory models, serving as examples of mental health, tackling problems realistically. Basically, they are supporting clients but more as 'side by side walkers'. All the plans, all decisions, all tasks – everything – is done together. Open interaction relations, the avoidance of authoritarianism and, in particular, mutual appreciation and the strengthening of self-esteem have characterized the communities. The principle of normality and living-learning in the everyday situations are important. Housework, jobs done for industry and other 'outsiders', and keeping one's room in order are a central part of activities. Besides these, group activities, creative work and various leisure activities are important.

Our research thus far carried out is not sufficiently deep to pinpoint the reasons why these communities have helped our clients so much. Hypotheses can, however, be proposed and the testing of these hypotheses is a task for our future research. The evolution of the hospitalization syndrome is naturally connected above all to the length of the hospital care period. The often-stiff regulations, limitations and hierarchy in the hospital ward together with the public attitude towards institutional care add to the susceptibility to hospitalization. A long-term patient starts to pick up features that e.g. Ludwig (1971) has described in his telling 'code' of chronicity. A model patient is dull, harmless and imperceptible – or, when he wants to draw attention he is aggressive or behaves in a queer manner. Characteristic also of part of this code are the avoidance of responsibility, the minimizing of stress, indifference towards other people, a black and white way of reacting, the right to unexpected behaviour and to some sort of diplomatic inviolability. Community care aims at releasing its clients from all of these.

We can assume that in small communities, the mobility of thoughts, feelings and activity linked to the interaction process may, to use Edelson's (1970) expression, release 'consolidated', patterned disturbances and prevent new ossifications. The models, norms and programmes jointly agreed upon within the group increase internal control. The group supports, feels, and responds to feelings: it is humane. The emerging security helps. The experience of human equality strengthens self-esteem, as does responsibility for the results of common and individual acts. The growth of self-esteem is the fundamental factor of all psychic rehabilitation. The group is as a family in which, at a more adult level and under guidance, delicate matters can be discussed and life experiences exchanged. It strives to teach its members to deal with new matters, to listen to other people, to defend oneself, to trust others, to accept and to resist. This learning process also gives more psychic manoeuvrability. The group's different objects of identification help them back to realities and to self-development. Community groups have shown how the relaxation of tension in interaction may often relieve internal psychic tension and distress at the individual level also.

Clear manifestations of community-level and individual development as described above can often only very slowly be found by close observation. Sometimes the improvement happens in a surprisingly short time. In traditional diagnostic terms, the clients may still be chronically ill persons, but their psychic state and level of socialization are quite different from the conditions pertaining during hospitalization which may have lasted for tens of years. Perhaps the most important change they have gone through is precisely their strengthened self-esteem and, accordingly, their greater capacity for independence and succeeding on their own.

This means that at least the vicious circle of hospitalization can be broken, that symptoms of institutionalization can be done away with. The experiments carried out by the Sopimusvuori Association have, as we see it, proved this unequivocally. Aware of the deep-rooted problems involved, we have come to the opinion that the activities described above could also to some extent prevent the very process of the making of a chronic patient, something that I tried to hint at on the hypothetical level earlier on. So our answer to the question in the chapter title is quite simply: yes.

The costs of Sopimusvuori rehabilitating activities compared with the corresponding hospital costs are clearly lower. Increasing personal autonomy, the importance of the new personal contacts created with the therapeutic community, improved possibilities for getting the patient's family to participate in the treatment process and a richer life in general are important factors. In these respects, a change from hospital-centred, more expensive care and rehabilitation towards less expensive forms of out-patient care is for most patients the only correct ethical solution (Vinni, Sillanpää & Anttinen, 1980).

As we also can see, the psychodynamic and social rehabilitation of persons with chronic schizophrenic disturbance still contains a lot of problems and many practical difficulties. We are in need of comprehensive longitudinal studies of the whole rehabilitation process. We need more research on the effects of interactions in egalitarian groups, the intentional activities, work and of the creative therapies which all seem to have a constructive influence on the personality, ego functions and especially on the self-esteem.

References

Anttinen, E. E., Eloranta, K. T. & Stenij, P. (1971). *Kotisairaanhoidon mahdollisuudet skitsofreniaa sairastavien jälkihoidossa ja kuntoutuksessa* (with English summary). Helsinki: Kansaneläkelaitoksen julkaisusarja A: 8.

Anttinen, E. E. & Jokinen, R. (1982). Kokemuksia Sopimusvuoren kuntoutuskotien toiminnasta (with English summary). *Sosiaalilääketieteellinen Aikakauslehti* **19**, 54–64.

Bleuler, M. (1972). *Die schizophrenen Geistesstörungen im Lichte langjähriger Kranken- und Familiengeschiechten.* Stuttgart: Thieme Verlag.

Brown, G. W., Bone, M., Dalison, B. & Wing, J. K. (1966). *Schizophrenia and Social Care.* London: Maudsley Monographs no. 17.

Ciompi, L. (1981). Wie können wir die Schizophrenen besser behandeln? Eine Synthese neuer Krankheits- und Therapiekonzepte. *Nervenarzt*, **52**, 506–14.

Ciompi, L. & Müller, C. (1976). *Lebensweg und Alter der Schizophrenen.* Berlin: Springer.

Edelson, M. (1970). *Sociotherapy and Psychotherapy.* Chicago & London: The University of Chicago Press.

Huber, G., Gross, G. & Schüttler, R. (1979). *Verlaufs- und sozialpsychiatrische Langzeitsuntersuchungen an den 1945–1959 in Bonn hospitalizierten schizophrenen Kranken.* Berlin: Springer.

Jones, M. (1968). *Beyond the Therapeutic Community. Social Learning and Social Psychiatry.* New Haven & London: Yale University Press.

Jones, M. (1978). *Maturation of the Therapeutic Community.* New York: Human Science Press.

Ludwig, A. M. (1971). *Treating the Treatment Failures.* New York: Grune & Stratton.

Moscher, L. R. & Keith, S. J. (1979). Research on the psychosocial treatment of schizophrenia: a summary report. *American Journal of Psychiatry*, **136**, 623–31.

Ojanen, M. (1978). *Hoito-ohjelmat ja Psykologiset Teoriat.* Tampere: Tampereen yliopiston psykologian laitoksen tutkimuksia 115.

Ojanen, M. (1980). *Yhteisöllisen Hoidon Lähestymistavat, Teoriat ja Menetelmät.* Tampere: Tampereen yliopiston psykologian laitoksen tutkimuksia 115.

Ojanen, M. & Saukkonen, P. (1975). *Tutkimus Sopimusvuoren toiminnasta.* Tampere: Kansanterveystieteen laitoksen julkaisusarja A, no. 15.

Vinni, K., Sillanpää, A. & Anttinen, E. (1980). Cost study of mental health services. In *Epidemiological Research as Basis for the Organization of Extramural Psychiatry*, ed. E. Strömgren, A. Dupont, J. Achton Nielson, pp. 258–64. Copenhagen: Munksgaard.

Wing, J. K. (1976). Eine praktische Grundlage für die Soziotherapie bei Schizophrenie. In *Therapie, Rehabilitation und Prävention schizophrener Erkrankungen*, ed. G. Huber. Stuttgart-New York: Schattauer.

Wykes, T. & Wing, J. K. (1982). A ward in a house: accommodation for 'new' long-stay patients. *Acta Psychiatrica Scandinavica*, **65**, 315–30.

Social network and the long-term course of mental disorders – research needs

H. KATSCHNIG AND T. KONIECZNA

Background

The study of the role of the social network in the course of mental disorders is a relatively new research challenge. The possibility of rehabilitating in the community mental patients who would otherwise spend their whole lives in psychiatric hospitals, has only emerged in the last few decades, mainly as a result of the introduction of neuroleptic drug treatment. Initially the concept of rehabilitation was, and in fact frequently still is, focussed on vocational rehabilitation; until recently, little attention has been paid to reintegrating a patient into his natural social environment.

The patient's social relationship in the community became an issue for research workers only after the phenomenon of 'revolving door psychiatry' had become apparent. The question was raised as to whether the early return of the mental patient to the psychiatric hospital was due to poor social integration or to life stress (Brown & Birley, 1968). However, the commonsense assumption that integration into a network of social relationships is an indicator of successful adaptation, since the support given by such relationships is protective, could only partially be substantiated (Henderson, 1983). It is true that having social relationships may reduce stress, strengthen the patient's ability to cope with stress or decrease the probability of relapse by enhancing the patient's compliance with medication; however, it is frequently overlooked that social connections make demands, create constraints, engender stress and impose pressure on one's opinions, attitudes and general life style (Hammer, 1981).

The study by Brown, Birley & Wing (1972; see also Vaughn & Leff, 1976) highlights the stressful aspects of social relationships: schizophrenic patients living in 'high expressed emotion' families had higher relapse rates than those living in 'low expressed emotion' households. Furthermore, while it is also true that the larger the number of social relationships the

Table 1. *Terms in the semantic field of 'social network'*

Neutral terms	Social contacts Social relations Social relationships Social connections Social context Social environment Social interactions
Terms stressing coherence or its contrary	Social coherence Social integration Social attachment Social support
	Social disintegration Loneliness

greater the possibility of a buffering effect of the social network in the face of adverse experiences, it is also true that a larger number of social relationships increases the possibility of life events associated with the disruption or distortion of network relationships.

Hence, this double-sidedness of social relationships has to be kept in mind when carrying out research in this field. A number of terms are employed in social psychiatric research for referring to the social relationships of patients, some of which are rather 'neutral', whereas others contain value judgments in that they either explicitly or implicitly stress the desirability of social relationships (see Table 1). Given the ambiguous nature of social contacts, it is advisable to use the neutral terms, of which the concept of 'social network' is one of the more promising and heuristically fruitful notions (Hammer, 1981).

The concept of 'social network'

The concept of 'social network' as a framework for describing an individual's social relationships has only recently been introduced by social anthropologists. In field studies social anthropologists have defined social network as 'a person's actual social relations that appear to be used and counted on by the individual' (Beels, 1978). A more concise definition describes the social network as 'the ways in which people are connected with each other' (Hammer, 1981).

It has been shown that each individual has a finite set of links between himself and others, which may come up to 1500 to 2000 relationships in a person's life (Mitchell, 1969), also including the indirect connections

Table 2. *Social sub-networks*

Home sub-network
Close family outside the home
Distant family outside the home
Close, best personal friends
Work/school connections
Neighbours
Organizational connections
Other friends or acquaintances
Professional caretakers

Source: Salzinger *et al.*, 1983

which link the initial (focal) individual to larger sets of people, such as friends of friends (Hammer, Makiesky-Barrow & Gutwirth, 1978).

The purpose of introducing the social network approach to social research was to have a more sophisticated tool for analysing social processes than the traditional social category variables (such as marital status or social class). It has also been suggested that the concept of social network could serve as a 'unifying framework' for interpreting research findings using the traditional social category variables (Mueller, 1980). Both the analytical concepts and the methods for eliciting information about social networks are still in a developmental stage.

The most basic approach to describing a social network is simply to count the number of social contacts within a given time period. These contacts can be categorized in terms of kin and non-kin relationships, or different sub-networks such as home sub-network, work connections, neighbours, etc. (Salzinger, Kaplan & Artemyeff, 1983; see Table 2).

Another way of analysing social network relationships is to take into account the degree of intimacy or psychosocial distance between persons who are related to one another. Five such 'zones' of intimacy may be distinguished (Boissevain, 1974; Pattison & Pattison, 1981):

1. *the personal zone:* persons with whom one lives and has high investment;
2. *the intimate zone:* persons of high psychosocial importance with whom one interacts frequently;
3. *the effective zone:* people with whom one interacts but who are less important; or important people with less interaction;
4. *the nominal zone:* people known, but of lesser importance and interaction;
5. *the extended zone:* people known about or linked through significant others.

Pattison & Pattison (1981) found that normal persons consistently and reliably named about 25 persons who were 'important' to them, which implied that the relationships were 'characterised by frequent interaction, positive affect, intense affect, a strong instrumental component of assistance, and balanced reciprocity of affective and instrumental exchange between ego and others'.

Describing social relationships in terms of their degree of intimacy or closeness is just one possible way of evaluating their quality, which can also be assessed on a number of other dimensions. For instance, the 'content' of a relationship may be described as an exchange of affect, of information or of material goods. Other concepts characterizing the quality of a relationship include the notions of reciprocity (exchange in both directions) and multiplexity (relationships having more than one 'content' area), both of which have been used in research on psychiatric patients (Tolsdorf, 1976; Sokolovsky *et al.*, 1978).

Finally, social networks may be described in terms of their structural characteristics, one aspect of which is 'configuration', i.e. the 'multi-dimensional geometry of the network' (Hammer, 1981). Examples of such configurations are (*a*) a hub, (*b*) a chain, and (*c*) a completely interconnected set (Hammer, 1981; see also Fig. 1). Size (number of members of the social network), density (proportion of the number of existing relationships compared to the number of all possible relationships) and frequency of contact are further examples of dimensions used for describing social networks. Unfortunately, the terminology is still very inconsistent in this field.

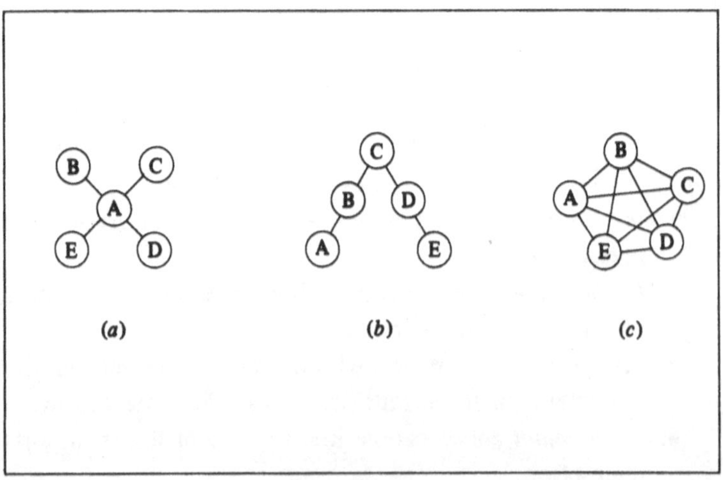

Fig. 1. Examples of network structures (after Hammer, 1981). (*a*) Hub, (*b*) chain, (*c*) completely interconnected set.

The uses of social network variables in research on the long-term course of mental illness

For the purpose of identifying research needs, it seems appropriate to distinguish three different uses of social network variables in studying the long-term course of mental illness.

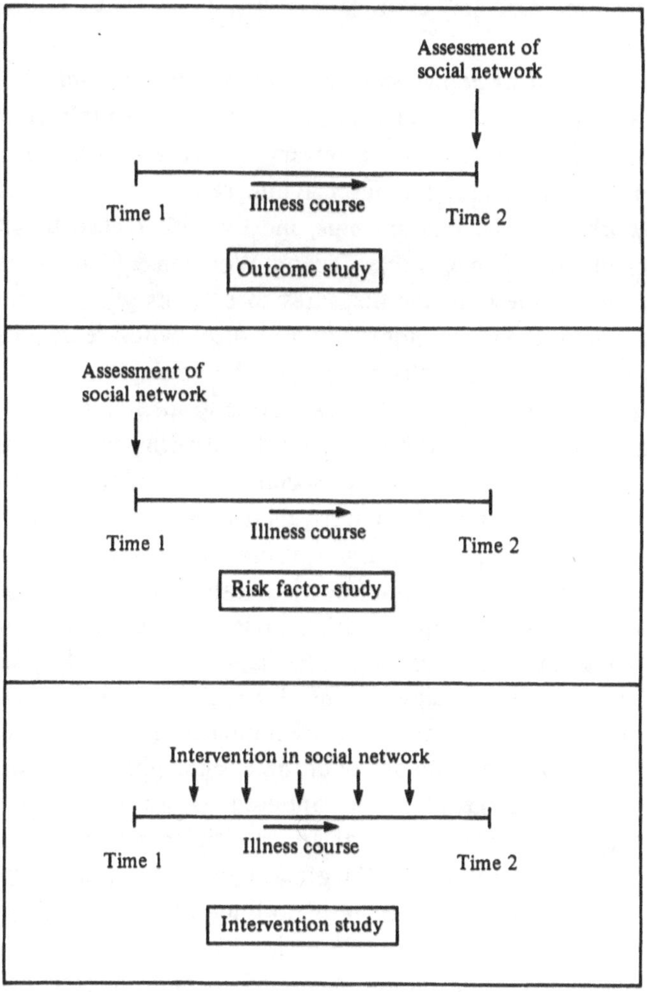

Fig. 2. Uses of social network variables in research on the long-term course of mental illness.

Social network variables have been employed in outcome studies where social category variables such as marital or employment status are taken into consideration. A second possible research use of social network variables consists in studying their role as risk factors for the occurrence of relapses or the development of an unfavourable course of psychiatric disorders. Finally, social network variables may be used explicitly as therapeutic factors in intervention/prevention studies.

Each of these three research uses of social network variables will be discussed in turn. However, it has to be stressed that this distinction is to some degree arbitrary and that a considerable overlap between these three types of research uses may exist.

The use of social network variables in outcome studies

Assuming that a specific social outcome is desirable in the course of psychiatric disorders is highly arbitrary. The concept which has usually been applied in this field is that of social integration, i.e. the reconstruction of a network of social relationships, mostly with regard to marital or occupational status. For example, Tsuang, Woolson & Fleming (1979) give the most favourable outcome measures to patients who are married or widowed, live in their own homes, and to those who are employed. The least favourable outcome is characterized by being single, living in a mental hospital and being incapable of working due to mental illness.

Wheras Tsuang *et al.* (1979) distinguish between good, fair and poor outcome, research workers using the social network approach describe the actual living situations of chronic psychiatric patients in more 'neutral' terms. Although such studies are not primarily concerned with outcome, they do in fact contribute to our knowledge about outcome by describing the social networks of chronic psychiatric patients, mostly of schizophrenic patients living in the community (e.g. Pattison *et al.*, 1975; Tolsdorf, 1976; Sokolovsky *et al.*, 1978; Lipton *et al.*, 1981; Pattison & Pattison, 1981). The findings of these studies are roughly comparable: in contrast to normal or neurotic samples the network of chronic schizophrenics is consistently smaller; the percentage of kin as opposed to non-kin relationships is higher; there are fewer reciprocal and multiplex and more dependent relationships than in samples of the general population; the network often includes persons with whom there is no long-term relationship; chronic schizophrenic patients have a rather peripheral position in their networks, their relationships being largely mediated through another individual; finally, the networks of schizophrenic patients contain many persons who are themselves mentally ill.

The difficulties inherent in this type of research are shown by the discrepant findings concerning the 'density', i.e. the interconnectedness, of the networks of chronic schizophrenics. While Pattison *et al.* (1975) found a higher density in the (smaller) networks of schizophrenic patients, Sokolovsky *et al.* (1978) did not discover any differences in network density between psychotic and non-psychotic residents of single-room-occupancy hotels. This discrepancy probably results from the fact that Sokolovsky *et al.* (1978) exclude, whereas Pattison *et al.* (1975) include, kin contacts in their measure of density (Mueller, 1980).

It is not clear from such cross-sectional descriptions whether these abnormal network characteristics of chronic schizophrenic patients are functional or dysfunctional, i.e. whether they correspond to the reduced level of social functioning of chronic patients and thus enable them to lead a satisfying life despite their disabilities, or whether these network characteristics themselves contribute to the disease taking an unfavourable course. The commonsense assumption that having an extensive social network with many close relationships is correlated with a person's psychological well-being may not be valid for chronic schizophrenic patients with their specific vulnerabilities. A possible answer to this question can only be obtained by conducting longitudinal studies which examine the course of the illness under different social network conditions.

The use of social network variables in risk factor studies

The concept of 'risk factor' is generally used in medical epidemiology to identify variables, the presence of which increases the risk of development of specific diseases (MacMahon & Pugh, 1970). Thus, heavy smoking is a risk factor for the development of pulmonary cancer, in the same way that the occurrence of loss events in a person's life increases the probability of his developing depression (Paykel, 1978), which is in turn increased by the lack of an intimate relationship (Brown & Harris, 1978).

We are not concerned here with the contribution of risk factors to the *development* of psychiatric disorders (e.g. Katschnig *et al.*, 1983), but with their contribution to the occurrence of *relapse* and the development of *chronicity*.

Little is in fact known about the role of social network characteristics in the course of mental disorders. Wing & Brown (1970) showed that, among other factors, reduced contact with staff and with the outside world contributed to the development of chronicity and negative symptoms in hospitalized psychiatric patients. The study by Brown *et al.* (1972) on the role played by 'high expressed emotion' in families of schizophrenic patients in the occurrence of relapse is another example (see also Vaughn & Leff, 1976, and Leff's chapter in this volume, pp. 241–5).

Sokolovsky *et al.* (1978; see also Cohen & Sokolovsky, 1978) studied the social networks of schizophrenic patients living in a single-room-occupancy hotel in New York City, relying not only on the patients' reports but also on their own observations of social interaction. They were interested in identifying factors which contribute to psychiatric rehospitalization. As expected, the severity of psychopathological symptoms was correlated with rehospitalization. However, the authors were also able to show that patients with small non-multiplex networks with low density run higher risks of rehospitalization than schizophrenics with more complex and extensive networks. Thus, it seems appropriate to conclude that chronic schizophrenics who are able to increase the size of their networks and become more involved in social life have a better chance to avoid rehospitalization. A more detailed analysis revealed that these social network characteristics were much more important for the rehospitalization of patients with minimal symptomatology than for the more severely ill.

These few studies show the possible usefulness of longitudinal studies for identifying social network risk factors which contribute to an unfavourable course of schizophrenia. As it is cumbersome to conduct such studies on a strictly prospective basis, it is tempting to collect social network information retrospectively. However, it has to be stressed that it is difficult in retrospective designs to disentangle the relationships between social network variables and psychopathology. As opposed to the study by Brown *et al.* (1972), which is a prospective study on the role of the quality of social network relationships for relapses, the investigation by Sokolovsky *et al.* (1978) is retrospective in design. Consequently, the authors raise the possibility that 'the data suggests that the patients' social network acted to obviate readmission, but it can also be argued that the rehospitalisation somehow resulted in a reduced network size'.

The risk factor concept may both be applied in naturalistic studies, i.e. in studies just documenting the course of psychiatric disorders under different social conditions, or in intervention studies. In the latter type of study, e.g. in trials of the long-term effect of psychotropic drugs on psychiatric disorders, social network variables should be taken into consideration as 'intervening factors', i.e. as factors which either increase or decrease the possible effect of the treatment method under study.

The use of social network variables in intervention/prevention studies

Once characteristics of the social network of chronic psychiatric patients have been identified which may act either as a risk or as a protective factor in relapse or chronicity, attempts can be made to change these network characteristics accordingly. We should like to suggest the following classification of intervention strategies which, in the context of our topic, may be regarded as strategies of tertiary prevention (i.e. prevention of relapse and chronicity). These strategies are not mutually exclusive and it may in fact be advisable to combine several of them for specific purposes. The proposed classification, however, serves as a guideline for planning interventions regarding the social network of chronic psychiatric patients.

1. *Correcting the existing social network* by (*a*) direct intervention (e.g. family therapy), or (*b*) indirect intervention (e.g. educating relatives, therapy for relatives).
2. *Expanding the existing social network* by (*a*) 'mobilising' (additional) family members, (*b*) putting relatives in touch with relatives of other patients (e.g. self-help groups) or (*c*) providing the possibility of additional social contacts for the patient (e.g. day-hospital, patient clubs, visiting nurse).
3. *Providing an alternative social network* by (*a*) transitional (e.g. half-way house) or (*b*) permanent (e.g. hostel).

Three types of intervention are distinguished: correcting the existing social network, expanding the existing social network and, finally, providing an alternative social network.

Strategies for correcting the existing social network include both classical family therapy and more pragmatic family therapeutic approaches (Gurman & Kniskern, 1981). For example, Falloon *et al.* (1982) were able to show in a controlled study that a specific form of goal-oriented behavioural family management prevented exacerbations in chronic schizophrenic patients. An indirect form of correcting the existing social network focusses on work with the relatives (e.g. Anderson, Hogarty & Reiss, 1980; Goldstein & Kopeikin, 1981; Leff *et al.* 1982). It has to be admitted, however, that the theoretical links of these studies with social network theory are rather weak which is due to the fact that they have not originated within the social network research tradition. However, the study by Leff *et al.* (1982) deserves special mention insofar as it explicitly attempts to modify a specific qualitative aspect of the network relationship (expressed emotion; see the chapter by Leff in this volume).

Carrying out research on the second strategy, expanding the existing social network, is extremely difficult. Clinical experience suggests that expanding the social network both on the part of the relatives and the patient may prove to be a rewarding prevention strategy. As far as the relative is concerned, 'mobilising' family members who have 'disappeared' or who have shown any interest, may be as helpful as putting relatives in touch with the relatives of other patients. The success of self-help organizations underlines the possible fruitfulness of this approach (Beels, 1978; Katschnig & Sint, 1984). As far as the patient's social network is concerned, the strategy of providing the possibility of additional social contacts in day-hospitals, patients clubs or the like, seems promising in the light of time-budget studies showing that exclusive contacts with high expressed emotion relatives may be harmful (Vaughn & Leff, 1976).

Finally, the strategy of providing an alternative social network, i.e. an artificial therapeutic network, can be pursued. It could be as much an alternative to the isolation of mental patients living in the community or the very limited social networks which are possible in a mental hospital, as to a natural social network (e.g. the family), which has been judged as being too stressful for the patient to continue living there. Such alternative networks can be provided on a transitional (e.g. half-way house) or a permanent (e.g. hostel or other sheltered living conditions) basis. They may be specifically geared toward the particular disabilities and requirements of patients. Mosher, Menn & Matthews (1975), Beard, Malamud & Rossman (1978) and Budson & Jolley (1978) provide examples of this strategy. It has to be stressed that carrying out these types of studies is very costly in terms of time, energy and man-power and therefore few such investigations have been undertaken so far.

Conclusion

The social network approach to studying the long-term course of illness in psychiatric patients is very promising in many respects. However, there are still several substantial methodological issues which need to be resolved. One of them is how to obtain adequate information about the network of psychiatric patients, for restricting oneself to information obtained from the patient alone may not be appropriate, given that the perception of others by mentally ill individuals is frequently distorted. Collecting information from additional sources, however, may be very costly. Another methodological problem consists in disentangling the complex relationships between social networks, psychopathology and other factors (such as neuroleptic drug therapy). At the same time, however, the influence of these other factors should be taken into consideration when studying social network aspects.

What is urgently needed are longitudinal studies which document changes in the social network and correlate such changes with the course of illness. We still do not know which type of social network, in terms of structure and quality, is decisive for a favourable long-term course of illness for specific groups of psychiatric patients.

Similarly as in other types of research on mental disorders, the way in which mental illnesses are defined in social network studies is of utmost importance. It is obvious that requiring cognitive disorders for diagnosing schizophrenia may yield different results in studies of social networks than using a definition of schizophrenia which allows this diagnosis in patients who are not thought-disordered (Berner *et al.*, 1983). Cognitive disorders seem to be especially deleterious for initiating and maintaining social relationships and the social networks of the latter group of patients may be quite different from those of the former due to their differing psychopathological characteristics.

In conclusion, it has to be underlined that many social-psychiatric and social-epidemiological research results which still seem to be inconsistent and isolated may, in fact, be more thoroughly understood by employing the framework of the social network. The social network approach, as a tool for analysing the complex process of interplay between the patient's disorder and his environment in more detail, could prove to be of crucial importance for really understanding the needs of the chronic mental patient.

References

Anderson, C. M., Hogarty, G. & Reiss, D. J. (1980). Family treatment of adult schizophrenic patients. *Schizophrenia Bulletin*, **6**, 490–505.

Beard, H. J., Malamud, T. J. & Rossman, E. (1978). Psychiatric rehabilitation and long-term rehospitalization rates: the findings of two research studies. *Schizophrenia Bulletin*, **4**, 622–35.

Beels, C. C. (1978). Social networks, the family, and the schizophrenic patient. *Schizophrenia Bulletin*, **4**, 512–21.

Berner, P., Gabriel, E., Katschnig, H., Kieffer, W., Koehler, K., Lenz, G. & Simhandl, Ch. (1983). *Diagnostic Criteria for Schizophrenic and Affective Psychoses*. Washington D.C.: American Psychiatric Press.

Boissevan, J. (1974). *Friends of Friends: Networks, Manipulators, and Coalitions*. New York: St Martin's Press.

Brown, G. W. & Birley, J. L. T. (1968). Crises and life changes and the onset of schizophrenia. *Journal of Health and Social Behavior*, **9**, 203–14.

Brown, G. W., Birley, J. L. T. & Wing, J. K. (1972). Influence of family life on schizophrenic disorders: a replication. *British Journal of Psychiatry*, **121**, 241–58.

Brown, G. W. & Harris, T. O. (1978). *Social Origins of Depression: A Study of Psychiatric Disorder in Women*. London: Tavistock Publications.

Budson, R. D. & Jolley, R. E. (1978). A crucial factor in community program success: the extended psychosocial kinship system. *Schizophrenia Bulletin*, **4**, 609–21.

Cohen, C. I. & Sokolovsky, J. (1978). Schizophrenia and social networks: ex-patients in the inner city. *Schizophrenia Bulletin*, **4**, 546–60.

Falloon, I. R. H., Boyd, J. L., McGill, C. W., Razani, J., Moss, H. B. & Gilderman, A. M. (1982). Family management in the prevention of exacerbations of schizophrenia: a controlled study. *New England Journal of Medicine*, **306**, 1437–40.

Goldstein, M. J. & Kopeikin, H. S. (1981). Short- and long-term effects of combining drug and family therapy. In *New Developments in Interventions with Families of Schizophrenics*, ed. M. J. Goldstein, pp. 5–26. San Francisco: Jossey-Bass.

Gurman, A. S. & Kniskern, D. P. (1981). *Handbook of Family Therapy*. New York: Brunner/Mazel.

Hammer, M. (1981). Social supports, social networks, and schizophrenia. *Schizophrenia Bulletin*, **7**, 45–57.

Hammer, M., Makiesky-Barrow, S. & Gutwirth, L. (1978). Social networks and schizophrenia. *Schizophrenia Bulletin*, **4**, 522–45.

Henderson, A. S. (1983). Vulnerability to depression: the lack of social support does not cause depression. In *The Origins of Depression: Current Concepts and Approaches*, ed. J. Angst, pp. 106–19. Berlin: Springer Verlag.

Katschnig, H., Angst, J., Clayton, J., Gershon, E. S., Hautzinger, M., Helmchen, H., Henderson, A. S., Klerman, G. L., Möller, H.-J., Paykel, E. S., Roth, M., Weissman, M. M. (1983). Risk factors, group report. In *The Origins of Depression: Current Concepts and Approaches*, ed. J. Angst, pp. 385–403. Berlin: Springer Verlag.

Katschnig, H. & Sint, P. (1984). Zwischen Selbsthilfe und Expertenhilfe: Die Angehörigenvereinigung 'Hilfe für Psychisch Erkrankte' in Wien. In *Angehörigenarbeit und Angehörigenselbsthilfe in der Psychiatrie*, ed. M. C. Angermeyer & A. Finzen, pp. 46–52. Stuttgart: Enke Verlag.

Leff, J., Kuipers, L., Berkowitz, R., Eberlein-Vries, R. & Sturgeon, D. (1982). A controlled trial of social interventions in the families of schizophrenic patients. *British Journal of Psychiatry*, **141**, 121–36.

Lipton, F. R., Cohen, C. I., Fischer, E. & Katz, S. E. (1981). Schizophrenia: a network crisis. *Schizophrenia Bulletin*, **7**, 144–51.

MacMahon, B. & Pugh, T. F. (1970). *Epidemiology: Principles and Methods*. Boston: Little, Brown & Co.

Mitchell, J. C. (ed.) (1969). *Social Networks in Urban Situations*. Manchester: Manchester University Press.

Mosher, L. R., Menn, A. Z. & Matthews, S. M. (1975). Soteria: evaluation of a home-based treatment for schizophrenia. *American Journal of Orothopsychiatry*, **45**, 455–67.

Mueller, D. P. (1980). Social networks: a promising direction for research on the relationship of the social environment to psychiatric disorder. *Social Science & Medicine*, **14A**, 147–61.

Pattison, E. M., Defrancisco, D., Wood, P., Frazier, H. & Crowder, J. (1975). A psychosocial kinship model for family therapy. *American Journal of Psychiatry*, **132**, 1246–51.

Pattison, E. M. & Pattison, M. L. (1981). Analysis of a schizophrenic psychosocial network. *Schizophrenia Bulletin*, **7**, 135–43.

Paykel, E. S. (1978). Contribution of life events to causation of psychiatric illness. *Psychological Medicine*, **8**, 245–53.

Salzinger, S., Kaplan, S. & Artemyeff, C. (1983). Mother's personal social networks and child maltreatment. *Journal of Abnormal Psychology*, **92**, 68–76.

Sokolovsky, J., Cohen, J., Berger, D. & Geiger, J. (1978). Personal networks of ex-mental patients in a Manhattan SRO hotel. *Human Organization*, **37**, 5–15.

Tolsdorf, C. C. (1976). Social networks, support and coping: an exploratory study. *Family Process*, **15**, 407–17.

Tsuang, M. T., Woolson, R. F. & Fleming, J. A. (1979). Long-term outcome of major psychoses. *Archives of General Psychiatry*, **36**, 1295–1301.

Vaughn, C. E. & Leff, J. P. (1976). The influence of family and social factors on the course of psychiatric illness: a comparison of schizophrenic and depressed neurotic patients. *British Journal of Psychiatry*, **129**, 125–37.

Wing, J. K. & Brown, G. W. (1970). *Institutionalism and Schizophrenia*. Cambridge University Press.

III: PUBLIC HEALTH ASPECTS OF LONG-TERM TREATMENT

Introduction to public health aspects of chronic illness and long-term treatment

H. HÄFNER

Problems of magnitude

In 1981, a group of World Health Organization (WHO) experts wrote in a booklet entitled *Social Dimensions of Mental Health*:

> There is a pressing need to deal with the consequences of... falling death rates in early life and increasing expectancy of life at birth; these paradoxically contribute to an increase in the prevalence of certain health problems. Among the most important of these consequences is the rising pandemic of chronic ill health and disability. (WHO, 1981)

In fact, life expectancy at birth has been increasing in most European countries from about 40 to 50 years in 1900 to 70 and more in 1980. A rapidly increasing part of our population reaches old age. Morbidity in general and prevalence of chronic illness in particular considerably increase in old age.

Problems of incidence

In addition to the greater proportion of the elderly afflicted by chronic illnesses or among chronically ill people, other factors also contribute to the same kind of health problem. The main age at risk for the onset of functional psychosis (the most frequent and severe mental disorders in adults), is about 20–34 years for schizophrenia and 24–50 years for affective psychoses. Given stable, age-related incidence rates, the total number of onsets of these disorders reflects the number of people reaching the ages at risk.

In some European countries, e.g. in the Federal Republic of Germany, the annual birth figures nearly doubled between 1945 and 1965. Then the annual birth figures fell steeply within five years to approximately half the number reached in 1964 and have been maintained at this level. As a consequence of these demographic changes, the Federal Republic is being confronted with a proportional increase in onsets of schizophrenia during the period 1975–2000 and can expect a proportional decrease thereafter. The same will presumably happen (albeit with a small time lag) with the figures for the true incidence of affective psychoses. The question still remains unanswered, whether – in addition to the demographic influence on the morbidity risk – the age-related incidence rates for depression have also been increasing and will continue to do so. At the time when the demographically determined morbidity figures presumably reach their peak, we may have reduced the number of psychiatric beds considerably and thus will not be able to serve the increased need.

Problems of prevalance

In the European countries, at all ages, life expectancy of people with primary handicaps, chronic illnesses and disabilities has increased much more than has the life expectancy of the total population. The reason for this is that medicine has succeeded in preventing and treating infectious and other acute fatal diseases. 'Techniques for preventing chronic illnesses have advanced much less rapidly than techniques for delaying death', as was reported by the WHO expert group on social dimensions of mental health (WHO, 1981).

In the field of mental health, the increase in life expectancy due to a reduction in premature death is most marked in mental retardation and dementia and less distinct in functional psychoses. When tuberculosis was almost eradicated in Europe between 1950 and 1970, one of the major causes for premature death of schizophrenics was removed. At present, people suffering from functional psychoses and particularly from schizophrenia may expect – after onset – half a century of life with recurring episodes of illness or with a lasting disability. Long duration of mental diseases or disabilities due to longevity also contribute considerably to prevalence figures and to the need for long-term medical care and social support.

One conclusion I would like to draw from this estimation of morbidity trends is that planners should observe demographic changes and keep some flexibility in the provision of services.

Changes in the health care policy

The drastic changes in the age structure and morbidity of the population in the European countries have brought with them a distinct change of the tasks to be fulfilled by a physician in particular, especially in primary health care; it has also effected a clear change in the functions of mental health services as a whole. In the developing countries, comparable changes have begun and might take a similar course in the future. The treatment of infectious and other acute diseases which end in healing or death (as was the case in the last century, when more than half of the deaths in European countries were caused by infectious diseases) is less and less at the focus of medical action. Instead, the long-term treatment of chronic diseases has come to the fore. The latter often requires long-term medication and careful control of effects and side-effects, prevention of undesirable sequelae or secondary phenomena and, last but not least, support of the chronically ill or disabled for coping with their long-term life problems.

Long-term diseases or disabilities in differing degrees affect the ability to work and to make contact, the social competence and – in severe cases – also the ability to arrange life independently. Functional psychoses in general and schizophrenia in particular, especially when taking a chronic course and having led to lasting impairments, frequently have unfavourable effects on the ability to work, on social competence, and on mental well-being. They not only burden the patient with a sense of a depressive or apathetically resigned reaction to the disease (which even aggravates the symptoms); they often also burden the family and the network of social relations by which a person is given support and protection on a biological and social level. Health care for the chronically ill in general and for frequently relapsing or chronic functional psychoses in particular requires measures complementary to the medicobiological treatment (e.g. drug maintenance, lithium prevention, etc.): psychological aids for coping with the disease, training of impaired mental and social abilities, and (if necessary) assistance in social and professional reintegration, as is stated in the chapters by Daly, Vaglum, Ciompi, and Anttinen in this volume.

Changes in mental health care policy

Beyond minor changes like the prevention of general paralysis or the implementation of psychoanalysis into psychiatry, two major shifts in mental health care policy took place within the last 100 years. The first was the filling up of large mental hospitals, which were isolated from general medicine, with chronic mental patients, mainly by compulsory admission (as noted by Daly and other contributors). Certainly, this system was not explicitly based on the results of empirical research. It turned out to have had at least a few shortcomings. During the last 25 years, we have shifted away from this system and taken more or less rapid steps in the opposite direction, towards the comprehensive community mental health care system. So far, the new policy is based only to a rather limited extent on research findings. These include the evaluation of rehabilitation programmes (e.g. Wing & Giddens, 1959; Wing, 1960; Bennett, Folkard & Nicholson, 1961, and others). One of the principles of the new philsophy of mental health care is the provision of alternatives to hospital care and of a network of various and differential facilities offering treatment and social support, especially for schizophrenic patients (as discussed by Ciompi and Anttinen in this volume). Some important questions concerning the advantages and the disadvantages of the new system as a whole and part of its newly introduced facilities remain unanswered. I shall mention only two:

1. It seems to be more difficult to control the standard of treatment and living conditions in numerous small institutions than in a few large mental hospitals. It cannot be denied that the standard of mental hospitals went rather out of control in the past. What is likely to happen with hostels and sheltered workshops for mental patients as time goes on? This seems to be mainly a question of practice, but Kushlick (1973) showed that it is possible to assess the characteristics of small institutions for the mentally retarded and to evaluate their work in a reliable way.
2. Up to the present we do not yet know, what group of schizophrenic patients really benefits from what part of the complex network of services offered to them. As has already been pointed out many times, we should especially promote evaluative research in this field.

Evaluation of community mental health services

A considerable number of studies evaluating the implementation and some outcome variables of community mental health services were based on an instrument that is powerful for monitoring the changing patterns of mental health care: the psychiatric case register. Studies based on case register data were carried out for example by Strömgren *et al.* (1979) and Dupont (1979) in Denmark, by Wing & Hailey (1972) in London, Fryers (1979) in Salford, and Torre, Marinoni & Allegri, (1982) in Lomest. But such registers rely on information from mental health services. They usually miss patients with primary care services, with social services, and with self-help groups. They also miss an important indicator of the effectiveness of a mental health care system: information about patients who drop out of contact with the mental health care services.

A methodology for supplementing case register studies should therefore be developed in order to get more complete information about the utilization of all mental health care services provided for patients with chronic functional psychoses and disabilities effected by these diseases. One possibility would be to collect information from the patients themselves in an economic way and to make a quantitative flow chart of services used, as proposed by Priest (this volume). Such a flow chart might enable us to identify patterns and pathways of utilization through the entire network of the care system. It might also provide quantitative measures which, for example, may be used as a basis for direct cost accounting. This methodology can be applied especially for evaluating the utilization of services by patients suffering from functional psychoses and other chronic mental disorders and for evaluating the effectiveness of care provided for them. Thus, it might also lead to an analysis of cost-effectiveness.

References

Bennett, D. H., Folkard, S. & Nicholson, A. (1961). Resettlement unit in a mental hospital. *Lancet*, **2**, 539–41.

Dupont, A. (1979). Psychiatric case registers. In *Estimating Needs for Mental Health Care*, ed. H. Häfner, pp. 43–51. Berlin, Heidelberg, New York: Springer.

Fryers, T. (1979). Estimation of need on the basis of case register data. In *Estimating Needs for Mental Health Care*, ed. H. Häfner, pp. 52–63. Berlin, Heidelberg, New York: Springer.

Kushlick, A. (1973). Evaluation of residential services for mentally retarded children. In *Roots of Evaluation*, ed. J. K. Wing & H. Häfner, pp. 175–96. London, New York, Toronto: Oxford University Press.

Strömgren, E., Kyst, E., Ryberg, I. & Weeke, A. (1979). Estimation of need on the basis of field survey findings. In *Estimating Needs for Mental Health Care*, ed. H. Häfner, pp. 37–42. Berlin, Heidelberg, New York: Springer.

Torre, E., Marinoni, A. & Allegri, G. (1982). Lomest psychiatric case register: old and new long-stay patients. *Social Psychiatry*, **17**, 125–31.

Wing, J. K. (1960). A pilot experiment on the rehabilitation of long-hospitalised male schizophrenic patients. *British Journal of Preventive and Social Medicine*, **14**, 173–80.

Wing, J. K. & Giddens, R. (1959). Industrial rehabilitation of male chronic patients. *Lancet*, **2**, 505–7.

Wing, J. K. & Hailey, A. M. (1972). *Evaluating a Community Psychiatric Service.* London: Oxford University Press.

World Health Organization (1981). *Social Dimensions of Mental Health*. Geneva: WHO.

Evaluation of long-term community care for patients with schizophrenia

H. HÄFNER AND W. AN DER HEIDEN

In the past a patient with a chronically disabling psychiatric illness such as schizophrenia has been treated by hospitalization lasting years or, often, a lifetime. Nowadays the trend has been to shorten hospital stay markedly and to continue treatment in the community through aftercare or the use of complementary services.

A main factor that has influenced the movement to treat the chronically disabled in the community rather than in the hospital has been clinical evidence of the debilitating effects of long-term institutional care. The treatment of chronic illness should focus upon helping patients to normalize their lives to the greatest possible degree and to raise their level of functioning; this is a role which the remote psychiatric hospital in particular can hardly fulfill. Whereas the development of drug therapy has encouraged the shift from hospital to community care, there is only a crude understanding of the forces in the community that help contain psychotic behaviour and help maintain the psychotic at a reasonable level of functioning.

Attkisson *et al.* (1978) pointed out, viewed from the perspective of the individual client a good care-giving system is one that does more than simply reduce a single problem or increase some restricted level of positive functioning. A good service must also be readily available when needed and operate in a fashion that does not create undue burdens for the consumer.

In practice, it is frequently observed that many persons seeking services have multiple problems and may therefore require simultaneous or well-integrated sequential treatments. Criteria for evaluating the effectiveness and adequacy of psychiatric care must therefore include a measure of programme continuity; this means coordination between services or, at least, of the degree to which a client can be referred from one institution to another.

Since 1969, a comprehensive community mental health service has gradually been set up in Mannheim, an industrial city with about 310000 inhabitants. Complementary services have been opened step by step according to need. On 1 January 1982, the complementary services comprised 3 homes providing 110 places and 4 sheltered apartments with 27 places; that is a total of 137 sheltered places for mentally ill persons (not counting homes for the elderly or psychogeriatric patients). The provision of out-patient, crisis and emergency services as well as of hospital beds flexibly conformed to the need. In a former publication (Häfner and Klug, 1980), we reported on the utilization trends of various levels of care during the period of implementation of an extensive mental health service in Mannheim.

Aims and hypotheses

There were two questions for investigation. 1. What impact does a comprehensive community mental health service have on the care provided for chronic schizophrenics on the three main levels:

- beds in psychiatric hospitals,
- places in complementary services for mentally ill (sheltered homes, apartments, etc.), and
- utilization of services for out-patient care?

In particular, how much care has to be provided in the community for discharged schizophrenics and for chronic schizophrenic patients who are no longer hospitalized for long periods? 2. What are the effects of an extensive community mental health service on the life of these patients with respect to institutionalization, treatment and course of their disease?

Within the framework of these questions, we set out to check the following hypotheses:

1. The number of so-called 'new' schizophrenics who are still in need of long-term institutionalization increases more markedly in sheltered homes than in mental hospitals.
2. A more extensive extramural care reduces the probability of readmission for hospital treatment.

Material and Method

Our evaluation was based on two steps:

1. On an analysis of utilization data of the Cumulative Psychiatric Case Register at the Central Institute of Mental Health (CIMH) in Mannheim, recorded for the period 30 May 1973 to 31

December 1980. This register covers all contacts of the inhabitants of Mannheim with 26 mental health services.

2. On a cohort study among all inhabitants of Mannheim who had been admitted to mental hospitals in the period 1 October 1977 to 30 September 1978 and were given the diagnosis schizophrenia (an der Heiden, Klug & Scheel, 1980).

Results

In concurrence with the findings of Magnus (1967), Hailey (1974), Wing & Fryers (1976), Howat (1979), Talbot (1979), Babiker (1980), Häfner & Klug (1982), and Torre *et al.* (1982), a group of 'new' long-stay patients was found to accumulate even under the conditions of an extensive community mental health service. We compared two groups:

1. the so-called 'old' long-stay population, comprising 222 inhabitants of Mannheim who had been hospitalized for more than one year on 30 May 1973, and
2. the 'new' long-stay population, i.e. 99 patients accumulated in the period 30 May 1973 to 31 December 1977.

We found significant differences. Those patients who, under the conditions of a community mental health service, require hospital care for more than one year, are significantly older and have had more previous treatment episodes than the 'old' chronic cases (Häfner & Klug, 1982).

The composition by diagnostic groups (Fig. 1) shows that the schizo-

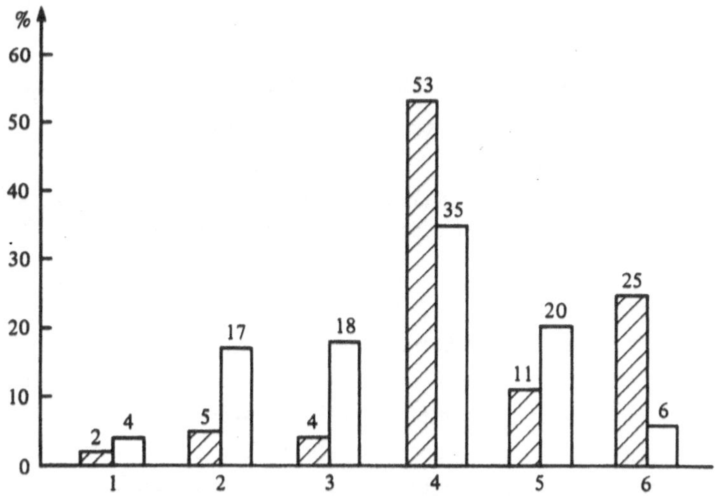

Fig. 1. Composition by six Diagnostic Groups. 1, Affective disorders; 2, neurotic & personality disorders; 3, alcohol & drug-related disorders; 4, schizophrenia & related disorders; 5, brain syndromes; 6, mental retardation. Hatched histograms, 'old longstays'; open histograms, 'new longstays'.

phrenics still make the largest contribution to the group of patients needing long-term hospitalization, although they have markedly decreased from 53% to 35%. The diagnostic composition and other characteristics of our group of long-stay patients, especially marital status and employment, are similar to the findings reported by Mann & Cree (1975), (see also Häfner & Klug, 1980, 1982).

Changes in the number of institutionalized schizophrenic cases or episodes, 1974–80

The total number of inhabitants of Mannheim with schizophrenia to whom care is provided in psychiatric hospitals and homes, reflects the heavy work load a mental health service still has to undertake for this diagnostic group, with its tendency to chronicity (Fig. 2).

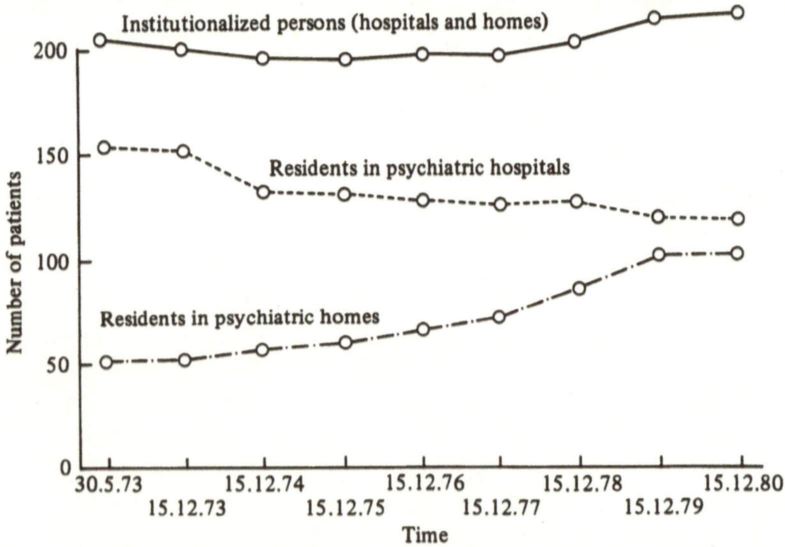

Fig. 2. One-day prevalences for care in psychiatric hospitals and homes provided for patients with schizophrenia (ICD 295) 1973–80.

In the following, a case is defined as any person living in Mannheim who has utilized a mental health service linked with the case register during the period of observation 1974–1980, whereas an episode means every admission of a patient to a mental health service.

The increase in treated episodes by about 50% and in the episode:case ratio 1.16 to 1.28 indicates that the frequency of readmission has increased over the period of observation (Table 1). The small rise in case numbers despite stable first-admission rates can be explained by an increase in discharged patients who are accommodated in complementary services or

Table 1. *Cases/episodes (ICD no. 295) in psychiatric institutions (hospitals, homes, etc.), 1974–80*

Year	1974	1975	1976	1977	1978	1979	1980
Cases	351	334	383	412	430	427	484
Episodes	407	389	447	487	535	559	621
Episode:case ratio	1.16	1.16	1.17	1.18	1.24	1.31	1.28

Table 2. *Length of stay of schizophrenic patients in psychiatric hospitals (treated episodes), 1974–80*

Length of stay (months)	1974	1975	1976	1977	1978	1979	1980
0–1	38[a]	43	71	90	88	94	146
	(23.2)	(25.0)	(31.3)	(35.3)	(31.7)	(32.6)	(38.2)
2–12	122	121	147	157	183	190	233
	(74.4)	(70.3)	(64.8)	(61.6)	(65.8)	(66.0)	(61.0)
12+	4	8	9	8	7	4	3
	(2.4)	(4.7)	(4.0)	(3.1)	(2.5)	(1.4)	(0.8)

Note: [a] Absolute frequency in each category for length of stay; percentage of yearly admissions in brackets.

are in need of further psychiatric care. This is an indicator of the growing density of the network of care.

Trends in the length of hospital stay

Correspondingly, the length of hospital stay of schizophrenic patients is markedly decreasing (Table 2).

The number of schizophrenics discharged within 1 month of hospital admission has risen significantly from 38 (23%) cases treated in 1974 to 146 (38%) in 1980. This reflects the increasing provision of short-term treatment of relapses, and of crisis intervention for patients with chronic mental illness who live in the community.

Trends in long-stay population of hospitals and homes, 1974–80

When the numbers of beds provided in hospitals and homes are combined, a slight increase of about 10% can be seen, as illustrated in Fig. 2. It results from a distinct increase of more than two-thirds in the numbers of patients institutionalized in complementary services and from a reduction of at least 30% in patients admitted to mental hospitals. This trend appears to be continuing.

The proportion of long-stay patients (over one year) among the total number of schizophrenics treated in psychiatric hospitals or homes (200–220) has declined from 192 (84%) on 30 May 1973 to 170 (74%) on 15 December 1980 (Fig. 3).

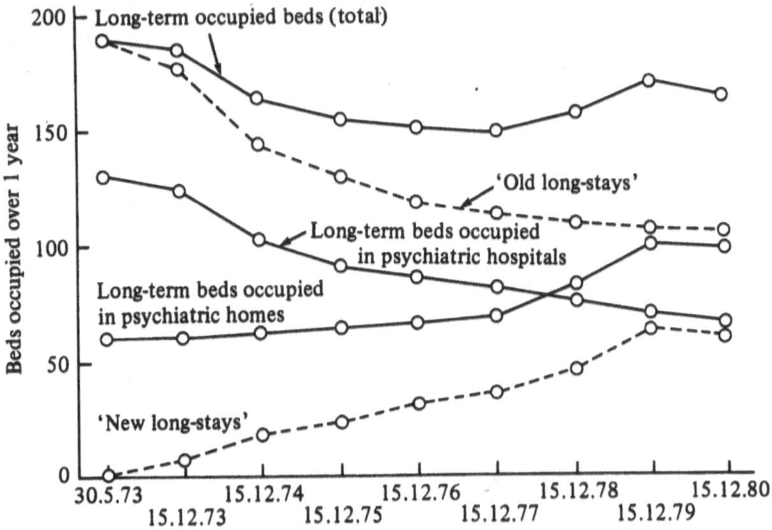

Fig. 3. Trends in 'old' and 'new' long-stay population (stay over one year) with schizophrenia, 1973–80.

Compared to the old-long-stay patients (census day 30 May 1973), whose numbers have continued to decline, even though more slowly, the new long-stay population has steadily accumulated over a period of 7.5 years, reaching 65 on 31 December 1980. While the number of beds in sheltered homes (including a facility outside Mannheim) providing psychiatric care for the Mannheim population has increased from 371 in 1973 to 443 in 1980, the over-proportional rise in schizophrenics admitted to sheltered homes is quite revealing. Within a period of seven years, this population has increased from about 30% to 60%. Three-quarters of those schizophrenics, who became long-stay patients in 1980 were admitted to homes, whereas one one-quarter were admitted to the psychiatric hospital.

These changes reveal that the main burden of institutional care provided for schizophrenic patients has shifted from the mental hospital to the community and to alternative mental health services (like sheltered homes, apartments, etc.). It seems that in the future, only one-quarter of those patients suffering from chronic schizophrenia and needing long-term institutional care will have to be placed in mental hospitals for more than 1 year.

Under the conditions of an effective community mental health service, the majority of this population can live in sheltered homes or apartments in the community. This shift brings with it far-reaching consequences for the organization of mental health services and for the extent of need for care.

In inquiring into changes in the extramural sector of care and also into factors and consequences influencing the outcome for patients, we observed the pattern of utilization by a group of 148 schizophrenic patients prospectively over a period of 18 months. The group consists of 148 Mannheim residents out of the total number of 195, who during 1 year (1 October 1977 to 30 September 1978) were admitted to a psychiatric hospital with schizophrenia and could be investigated over the whole period of observation. 47 could not be reached at all or not at every date of examination, because of death, removal or refusal. Admissions had been made to one of the three psychiatric hospitals serving Mannheim. A special record system (an der Heiden & Klug, 1980), which was developed for this study, gives more precise information on patient careers in a network of in-patient, out-patient and complementary services.

After an average length of stay of 91 days, the patients were discharged from the hospital treatment which had led to their inclusion into the sample. For 68 out of 148 patients, this remained the only hospital admission during the period of observation. 80 patients (54%) had been readmitted at least once; the peak was seven hospital stays within a period of 18 months (Fig. 4). The previous course of the disease has turned out

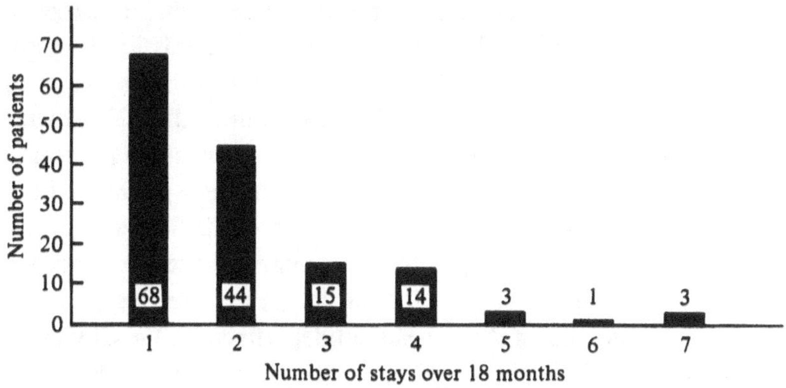

Fig. 4. Statistics of in-patient care. 1–7: Number of hospital stays during an 18 month period of observation. Average length of stay in hospital: 91 days; average interval between discharge and readmission: 170 days; average total of length of stay in psychiatric hospital per patient during an 18 month period: 144 days.

Table 3. *Rates of intra- and extramural care*

Institution	*n* (patients)	Average rate per 100 patients and year[a]
Psychiatric hospital	148	9270 days
Day- /night-hospital	6	284 days
Sheltered homes	38	4700 days
Sheltered workshops	36	2560 days
Psychiatric out-patient department	136	485 contacts
Psychiatrists in free practice		915 contacts
Other physicians		460 contacts
Patients' clubs and miscellaneous	67	245 contacts

Note: [a] The calculation of the rates is based on a total of 148 patients.

to be the most important predictor of the number of readmissions to in-patient services. The more previous in-patient treatments, the more frequently the patient has to be readmitted to hospital. ($r = +0.25$; $p < 0.001$) The average interval until readmission was 170 days for patients who had had several previous hospital stays.

Table 3 illustrates the utilization of in-patient, out-patient and complementary services by comparable rates (hospital days per 100 patients per year; contacts per 100 patients per year). The low number of patients staying in the day-hospital is mainly due to the fact that the only hospital of this kind serving the inhabitants of Mannheim at the time of investigation was situated in Heidelberg, 20 km away. 38 patients had lived in half-way houses or sheltered homes most of the time after their discharge from hospital. For 5 of these patients this was the first admission to a home. For 36 members of this patient group, care was provided in one of the 2 sheltered workshops located in Mannheim. They amount to 27% of a total of 126 patients who, according to their own statements, have remained unemployed. From the viewpoint of medical care, these figures make clear how smooth the transition is from hospital to out-patient aftercare. 136 of the schizophrenics discharged from hospital had been in contact with medical services. The majority of them (90%) had seen psychiatrists in practice or had contacted the out-patient department of the CIMH. 3 out of the remaining 12 patients could not be discharged during the 18-month period; 5 lived in sheltered homes and were provided with care by a psychiatric consultant. Only 4 patients had not been seen by any physician.

Attention should be paid to the fact that 25 patients of the group have been treated by several physicians simultaneously for periods of at least

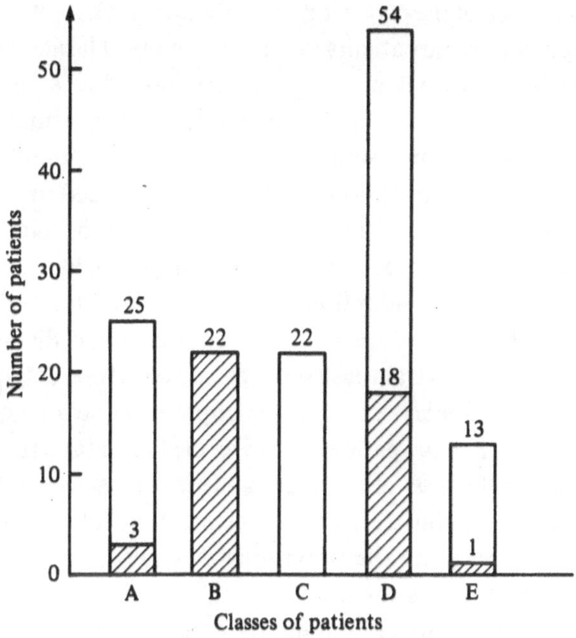

Fig. 5. Medical out-patient care provided to schizophrenic patients of Mannheim ($n = 136$). A, more than one physician at the same time; B, change between out-patient department, psychiatrist in practice, and family doctor; C, psychiatric out-patient department; D, psychiatrist in practice; E, family doctor. Hatched histograms indicate a change of doctor.

3 months (Fig. 5). This is due partly to the organization of the health care services in the Federal Republic of Germany. Patients receiving social insurance benefits must first consult a general practitioner, who decides whether or not they need specialist treatment. The referral has to be renewed every 3 months. Some of the patients actually take medical advice from both their family doctor and from a specialist over prolonged periods of time. This is a serious problem in relation to costs and to questions of patient compliance.

Roughly 30% of the patients have changed their physician at least once in the 18-month period and thereby interrupted the continuity of medical aftercare. This high proportion reflects the difficulties of schizophrenic patients in entering into trusting relations (Tantam & Klerman, 1979). These findings have made clear that extramural care is often not limited to the utilization of a single agency. Very frequently, patients contact several, in extreme cases up to five agencies at the same time. Most cases of multiple utilization consist of visits to a physician combined with stays in sheltered homes, attendance at a sheltered workshop or/and a patients' club. This is one consequence of the provision of a network of rehabilitation facilities for chronic schizophrenic patients in the community. The network provides various kinds of help depending on the individual's needs (medical treatment, housing, occupation and social activities). The number of hospital admissions before inclusion in the sample was found to correlate positively with the utilization of facilities provided in the community, as measured by the number of weeks spent out of hospital in which some form of aftercare was received ($r = +0.40$; $p < 0.0001$).

This trend indicates the flexible adaption of the network of social and medical care to the needs which arise from the course of the disease; however, the extent of use of extramural services varies. More detailed analysis shows that, given a similar course of schizophrenia and an equal number of hospital stays, female patients receive medical aftercare or contact services significantly less often than male patients ($r = 8.15$; $\mathrm{df} = 2$; $p < 0.02$). This may point to the fact that many female patients cannot make consequent use of all the provisions they need, because of their family, household and professional duties.

The essential aims of an extensive community care for schizophrenic patients are to prevent long-term hospitalization (Byers, Cohen & Harshbarger, 1978) and to enable the chronically mentally ill and disabled patients to live and participate in their normal surroundings as long as possible. In fact, the dense network of extramural services provided in Mannheim seem to have this effect.

We have divided the cohort into three subgroups by intensity of utilization, which was operationalized by summing up all contacts of a patient with extramural services during the stay outside hospital. On this basis, the whole sample was divided into three subgroups and the probability calculated for each that its members will not need hospitalization. The object of this analysis is to be able to predict the mean interval between discharge from an in-patient service and readmission (Fig. 6).

For the subgroup with the most extensive utilization of complementary services, the cumulative probability of not being readmitted to hospital within one year is 0.30. The probability for the subgroup with medium utilization, 0.14 is considerably lower. The subgroup with lowest utilization rates is not fully comparable, since it mainly consists of patients with a relatively short period since first admission and thereby a more favorable prognosis. From the difference between subgroup 2 and subgroup 3 in probability of getting readmitted we may conclude that an extensive utilization of extramural facilities reduces the risk of readmission to psychiatric hospital.

The pattern of utilization over time can be seen as a dynamic process

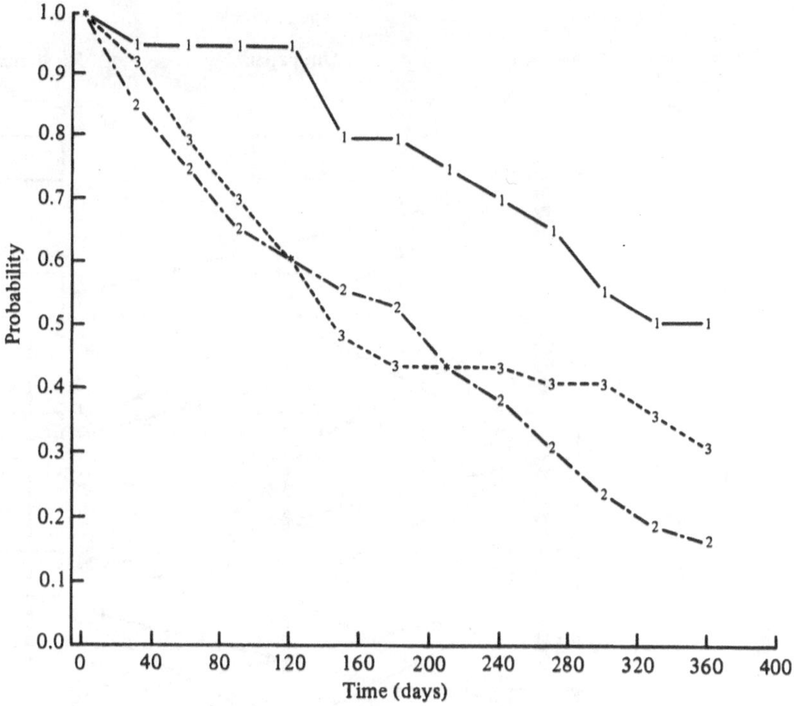

Fig. 6. Extramural care and probability of readmission.

which is reflected by the transition between the various states of care. In order to illustrate this process, we have made three categories of utilization according to the intensity of care:

- in-patient treatment;
- extramural aftercare;
- no aftercare.

The patient stream can now be clearly illustrated by means of a flow chart (Fig. 7). Analysis of the patient stream shows the transitions for all 148 patients. At cross-sectional point 1, all 148 patients are still in hospital. 14 days later, at point 2, 12 patients have been discharged; 10 of them have contacted an aftercare service and two have not received any aftercare; 136 patients remain in hospital. From cross-sectional point 3 on, the changes become more complex. One first readmission to hospital has been made from the 'aftercare' section. Furthermore, one patient who so far has not received psychiatric treatment, has changed over to the aftercare sector. Altogether, a distinct decrease can be observed in the in-patient sector, corresponding to a marked increase in the 'aftercare' and 'no aftercare' categories.

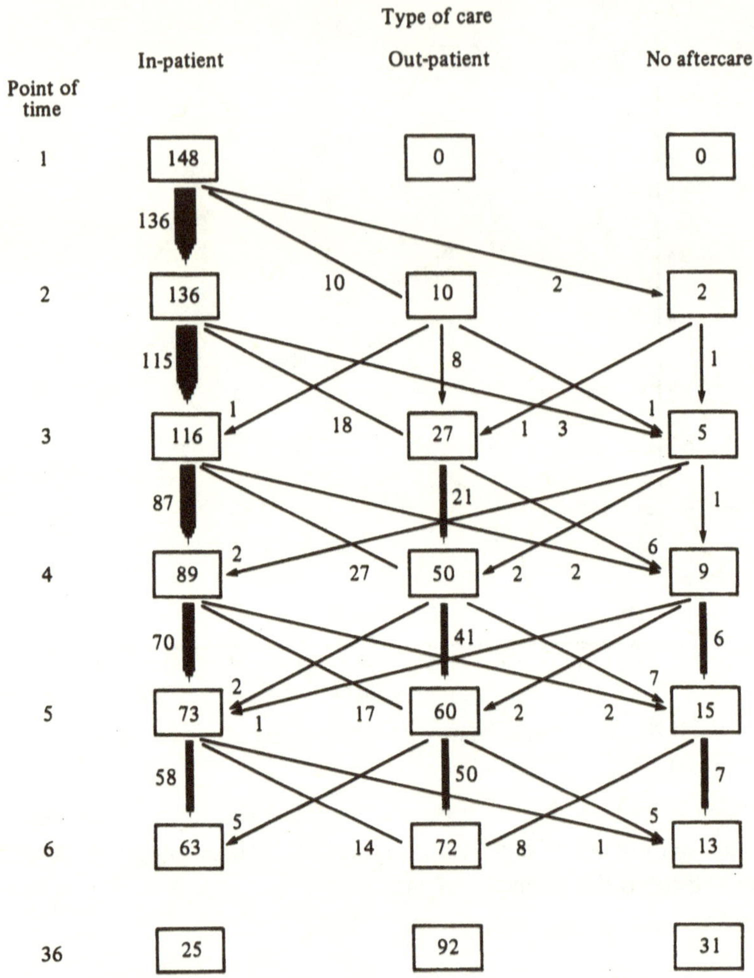

Fig. 7. Pathways through services.

Especially in planning psychiatric services to cover population needs the future pattern of utilization is a criterion of the utmost importance. The dynamics of the patient cohort, which are reflected in the transition from one category of care to another, may serve as a basis of forecasting future trends in the patient stream by applying more sophisticated statistical techniques such as, for example, time series analysis.

Discussion

The implementation of a dense network of complementary services for the treatment of schizophrenic patients brings with it a shift of the main burden of care from the mental hospital to complementary services in the community. While there have been a number of demonstrations of the effectiveness of alternatives to hospitalization (see for example Test & Stein, 1978), nowadays the economic motive plays a more and more important part in the provision of different systems or types of long-term treatment, rehabilitation and social support for patients with chronic functional psychosis.

Utilization data of the above-mentioned 148 patients with schizophrenia served as a basis for conducting a pure cost analysis. First results demonstrate that, compared with the costs for long-stay institutional care the use of a network of complementary services in the community is approximately half as expensive.

An overall aim of an economic survey of the psychiatric health care system is to study alternative uses of limited resources; that means that both the costs and the results must be measured at some level. A decision will be based upon the answer as to whether the total benefits exceed the total costs. As Weisbrod, Test & Stein (1980) pointed out, what is controversial is not whether benefits and costs should be compared but what to count as benefits and costs and how to compare them.

Another subject that needs more detailed and specific investigation than has been given so far, is that of the burden for the relatives. A considerable part of the success of a community care system depends upon the support for patients given by their relatives, who provide most of the domestic supervision that would otherwise be given by trained staff in hospitals of sheltered homes. The increasing number of short-term intramural treatment episodes per patient in our group may point to the necessity that more attention must be given to the social–psychological milieu to which a discharged patient must return in the community and to the conditions that might increase the probability of being able to remain there.

References

Attkisson, C. C., Hargreaves, W. A., Horowitz, M. J. & Sorensen, J. E. (eds) (1978). *Evaluation of Human Service Program*. New York–London: Academic Press.

Babiker, I. E. (1980). Social and clinical correlates of new long-stay. *Acta Psychiatrica Scandinavica*, **61**, 365–75.

Byers, E. S., Cohen, S. & Harshbarger, D. (1978). Impact of aftercare services on recidivism of mental hospital patients. *Community Mental Health Journal*, **14**, 26–34.

Häfner, H. & Klug, J. (1980). First evaluation of the Mannheim community mental health service. In *Epidemiological research as a basis for the organization of extramural psychiatry*, ed. E. Strömgren, *Acta Psychiatrica Scandinavica*, Suppl. 285, **62**, 68–78.

Häfner, H. & Klug, J. (1982). The impact of an expanding community mental health service on patterns of bed usage: evaluation of a four-year period of implementation. *Psychological Medicine*, **12**, 177–90.

Hailey, A. M. (1974). The new chronic psychiatric population. *British Journal of Preventive and Social Medicine*, **28**, 180–6.

Heiden, W., an der & Klug, J. (1980). An integrated record system for the observation of the demand for medical and social aftercare as basis for organizing extramural services.

In *Epidemiological Research as Basis for the Organization of Extramural Psychiatry*, ed. E. Strömgren, A. Dupont & J. Achton Neilson, pp. 54–9. Copenhagen: Munksgaard.

Heiden, W., an der, Klug, J. & Scheel, R. (1980). A cohort study of the use of aftercare facilities. In *8th International Congress on Health Records*, vol. 2, ed. J. Velthoven, pp. 344–63.

Howat, J. (1979). Nottingham and the hospital plan: a follow-up study of long-stay in-patients. *British Journal of Psychiatry*, **135**, 42–51.

Magnus, R. V. (1967). *The new chronics. British Journal of Psychiatry*, **113**, 555–6.

Mann, S. & Cree, W. (1975). The new 'long-stay' in mental hospitals. *British Journal of Hospital Medicine*, July, 55–63.

Talbot, J. A. (1979). Care of chronically mentally ill: still a national disgrace. *The American Journal of Psychiatry*, **136**, 688–9.

Tantam, D. & Klerman, G. (1979). Patient transfer from one clinican to another and dropping-out of out-patient treatment. *Social Psychiatry*, **14**, 107–13.

Test, M. A. & Stein, L. I. (1978). The clinical rationale for community treatment: A review of the literature. In *Alternatives to Mental Hospital Treatment*, ed. M. A. Test & L. I. Stein, pp. 3–22. New York/London: Plenum Press.

Torre, E., Marinoni, A. & Allegri, G. (1982). Lomest psychiatric case register: old and new long-stay patients. *Social Psychiatry*, **17**, 125–31.

Weisbrod, B. A., Test, M. A. & Stein, L. I. (1980). Alternative to mental hospital treatment. II. Economic benefit-cost analysis. *Archives of General Psychiatry*, **37**, 400–5.

Wing, J. K. & Fryers, T. (eds) (1976). *Psychiatric Services in Camberwell and Salford. Statistics from the Camberwell and Salford psychiatric registers 1964–1974*. Medical Research Council Social Psychiatry Unit, London and the Department of Community Medicine, University of Manchester.

Case registers for monitoring treatment outcome in chronic functional psychoses

D. WALSH

Introduction

A register is simply a collection of persons or things with common characteristics. Thus the Villa Lante, the Palazzo Farnese and the Palazzo Barberini are Italian buildings of architectural and aesthetic merit. They, therefore, may appear in a register or list of buildings worthy of preservation.

In a more medical context, cancer registers, registers of congenital malformations, twin registers and adoption registers have been established to further our knowledge of the incidence, prevalence and origins of disease.

Psychiatric case registers

Psychiatric case registers have the common characteristic that they gather information on persons who have received treatment for psychiatric illness. In practice, however, this usually means patients who have received treatment only by the psychiatric services. So psychiatric case registers do not include patients who have consulted general practitioners or other medical or social agencies because of psychiatric complaints, nor do they contain individuals who, although psychiatrically ill, have not contacted any services.

However, the title *case*-register has a specific connotation which goes beyond a mere listing of individuals. It implies the establishment of a continuing record of a person's contact with the psychiatric services once he has entered the network. The case register system must therefore accumulate over time longitudinal information on individual patient careers. Furthermore this longitudinal information can be obtained by a mechanism of *linking* the individual spells of contact of the same individual within the same service or between different services. The recognition of the same individual at multiple points of contact and at different periods of time is technically brought about by use of his personal number, in countries where this exists, or by other identifying data in sovereignties where no personal number exists. In this latter case, linkage will be dependent on the acquisition of accurate data on names, including maiden name in the case of married women who have changed their birth names, date of birth, place of residence and so on.

Another essential element of a case register is that it acquires information on individuals who live within a defined population or catchment area. All reasonable efforts are undertaken to obtain information on individuals resident in the catchment area but consulting services outside it. Some difficulties are experienced in some jurisdictions where private services operate as they are sometimes reluctant to give information on their clientele. An outstanding example of where this occurs is the United States of America.

Ideally a psychiatric case register should follow individual patient movements through all aspects of psychiatric care but some national registers confine their activities to in-patients only (examples are Denmark and Norway).

One example of a case register system which attempts to link information from psychiatric treatment sources to those of general hospital and other specialized hospital services is that of the Oxford record linkage project. Here an attempt to uncover significant relationships between psychiatric and other illnesses has not been particularly successful.

Psychiatric case registers currently operating in Europe

Among the countries represented at this workshop the following currently operate case registers.

The United Kingdom

1. The first psychiatric case register began operating from Mapperley Hospital, Nottingham, where it was established by the late Dr Duncan McMillan in 1960 (Department of Health and Social Security, 1971).
2. The Camberwell psychiatric case register, operated by the Institute of Psychiatry, was established in 1964 based on the population of the London borough of Camberwell of approximately 170000 (Wing & Fryers, 1976). Originally this register covered patients in all forms of psychiatric care. Recently however there has been a curtailment and in-patients only are included. However it is understood that the register will shortly be reverted to total psychiatric service coverage.

3. The Salford psychiatric case register has been operated since the 1960s by the Department of Community Medicine in the Manchester borough of Salford (Fryers & Wooff, 1974).
4. The Worcester psychiatric case register has been set up in an area where a policy of phasing out psychiatric hospitals at Powick has been undertaken.
5. The Southampton psychiatric case register (Grad de Alarcon & Nelson, 1974).
6. The Oxford psychiatric case register (Baldwin, 1974).
7. The Aberdeen psychiatric case register. This was an early register covering a population of approximately 500 000 people in northeast Scotland and based on Aberdeen. Here extensive socio-demographic information on individual patients is gathered by trained and experienced case register interviewers (Baldwin *et al.*, 1965). This is in contrast to most registers where information is gathered by the admissions or medical records office.
8. The Cardiff psychiatric case register.

In addition to these existing psychiatric case registers in the United Kingdom it is understood that the setting up of a further register at Edinburgh is being contemplated.

For some years now an attempt has been made in the United Kingdom to harmonize technologies and objectives in the case register field. To this end annual meetings under the auspices of the Department of Health and Social Security have been held. These have been taking place at two levels. The first level is that of medical directors of the case registers and the second is for the data processing managers responsible for each register. In this way a commitment to working towards standardization of practice has been established. Agreement has been reached on standardized output for common parameters. This enables comparisons to be made between registers.

Holland

The Groningen psychiatric case register in Holland provides extensive coverage for a population of about 40 000. It is operated by the Social Psychiatry Department at the University of Groningen (Giel & ten Horn, 1982).

Denmark

The Aarhus County psychiatric case register operated by the Institute of Psychiatric Demography at Aarhus operated during the 1970s but is not currently in action. However, the national Danish in-patient case register is operated by the Institute (Dupont, Videbech & Weeke, 1974).

Federal Republic of Germany

At Mannheim, Germany, a case register covering approximately 400000 people has been operated by the Central Institute for Mental Health of the University of Heidelberg (Häfner & Klug, 1982). This case register ceased operating on the intervention of the German data commissioner a few years ago. However the register has been allowed to keep existing data and has not been obliged to destroy them.

Italy

The Lomest psychiatric case register is operated by the psychiatric team at the University of Pavia (Torre, Marinoni & Allegri, 1982).

Switzerland

A psychiatric case register operates at Geneva covering a population of approximately 400000 people in the city and canton of Geneva.

Iceland

Iceland has long had an in-patient and extra-hospital psychiatric reporting system which is currently operating to a limited extent.

Ireland

In Ireland two psychiatric case registers operate and we shall be returning to these in a moment.

Data Protection Laws

Concern about the privacy rights of individuals in many human areas has been growing. With the expansion of electronic data processing and the possibility of holding personalized information on computer files there have been active movements to uphold the right to privacy. This has led to what are collectively called 'Data Protection Laws'. These have been taken to their furthest in the Federal Republic of Germany where a Data Commissioner has been established to investigate the activities of each and every personal data file. The consequence of this for the psychiatric scene is that the only psychiatric case register operating in Germany, that at Mannheim, has been forced to cease operation. However, there is hope that these restrictions will be relaxed and the register, which has been allowed to retain data already gathered, will be able to continue operations before too long.

Three general provisions govern the approach to civil rights in relation to electronically banked personal information. They are that the individual must give informed consent before any information is obtained from him, that he has the right of access to information held about him and, if believing the information to be incorrect, he has the right to have it changed. In the United Kingdom, proposed general legislation is likely to exempt psychiatric data sources from the second of these two requirements and to assume consent when individuals enter a treatment centre.

In other countries where no formal approach has yet been adopted to the problem it is likely that the judicial approach to such problems would be that conventional medical ethical behaviour in relation to patient's confidentiality be observed. However, these countries are likely to be affected by data protection legislation in the light of the Council of Europe resolution which member states will be asked to sign. It seeks to provide safeguards along the lines already indicated (Council of Europe, 1982).

Technical problems

A recent World Health Organization (WHO) meeting on 'Psychiatric Case Registers' at Mannheim embracing directors of several registers indicated the difficulties that the various parameters useful for comparison entail. Thus definitions such as those of prevalence, those of 'episodes of care' and spells of contact appear to differ significantly between various registers. In consequence comparability of output between different European registers still poses considerable problems. It is hoped that the Mannheim meeting will be the first in a series attempting to standardize definitions between registers and so harmonize output.

Registers and medical treatment

The limit of utility of a psychiatric case register for determining treatment outcome will depend on the extent to which the register incorporates medical treatment data. In essence this means the bringing together of routine socio-demographic and diagnostic material (gathered by all registers) and specific treatment data in the one file. Some registers are integral with the medical case record and therefore pose no difficulties in this matter. However probably the majority of registers have separate case register and medical record systems. In these cases the system of itself will offer no possibility of monitoring outcome in terms of service utilization coincidental with the specific medical treatment influences. For this to be done two systems will have to be operated and utilized individually.

The utility of a case register then is:

1. Treatment outcome may be monitored, as defined by service contact. This, of course, is a very limited achievement but more importantly the register can provide samples of individuals who

have undergone treatment; they can then be followed up for more specific purposes.

2. The register enables specific socio-medico-demographic interactions of a causal or influential nature on the course of psychiatric illness to be studied.
3. The register has, of course, enormous administrative uses in predicting future service needs and so helps the planning of psychiatric services. For example, registers have been able to tell us the number of patients becoming 'new long-stay' in various services and whether trends in the build-up of new long-stay patients are discernible. In the same way registers have shown that patients utilizing hostels often tend to become chronic or long-stay in this type of accommodation.
4. Registers can provide adequate and reliable out-patient data in situations where these data were previously unreliable.
5. Registers can provide the basic information to enable cost-effective and cost-benefit studies in the field of mental health to be undertaken.

The limitations of the register as a tool for measuring output have already been indicated. First they give information only on patients treated by the specialist psychiatric services. Second, in many cases they do not provide information on treatments received.

The Irish case registers

To illustrate the utility of psychiatric case registers in evaluating outcome I shall provide an illustration from my own country.

In Ireland, two psychiatric case registers operate. The first of these is called the St Loman's psychiatric case register. It covers the psychiatric service of this name catering for a population of approximately 250000. This is a new psychiatric service which operates with, by Irish standards, a very limited bed provision. There are 200 beds giving an in-patient bed ratio of 0.7 per 1000 of population.

The second register is called the Three County register. This covers three separate Irish services in three counties. The population, in contrast to the St Loman's service, is mainly a rural one and serves 150000 people. Here there is a much greater dependence on beds than in the St Loman's area; the overall bed ratio is 4.5 per 1000 of population.

In-patient data, which have existed since the late 1850s have clearly shown that the Irish in-patient hospitalization rate was the highest known (Walsh & Walsh, 1970). No clear light could be thrown on the reasons for this situation until the case registers came into operation. They have shown that Irish psychiatric services, by comparison with those of other areas where case registers are operating, have much higher prevalence rates. Thus the excess of patients is not merely a hospital affair. Out-patient services also show high prevalence rates. It is also clear that rates of contact of persons beginning new episodes of care with Irish registers is significantly lower than in other register areas. Thus the general picture of Irish psychiatric services made clear by registers is that patients contact psychiatric services less frequently but once they enter the psychiatric network are less likely to leave. Thus patients find it difficult to enter psychiatric care in Ireland but once in are more likely than elsewhere to remain there.

Prevalence rates

The high prevalence rates in Ireland may be exemplified by pointing out that the St Loman's register gives one-day prevalence rates that are slightly higher than those of Camberwell, thus the one-day prevalence rate in this area of population aged 15 and over for all illnesses is 1%. For schizophrenia it is 0.3% and for neuroses it is also 0.3% (Walsh, Butler & Starks, 1981). In the Three Counties however, the prevalence rates are considerably greater. The rate for all diagnoses is 2% of the population aged 15 and over, for schizophrenia 0.8% and for neuroses 0.45% (Walsh *et al.*, 1980).

That these prevalence rates, in the case of the Three Counties, are not artefacts of diagnosis has been confirmed by the Medico-Social Research Board study (niNualain *et al.*, 1984). This project involved the residence of a psychiatrist and social researcher in each of the three counties for 1 year, serially. The psychiatrist had been trained in the use of the Present State Examination. This was administered to every prevalence patient given a diagnosis of schizophrenia. The researcher also examined all new cases of alleged schizophrenia contacting the services; this will be the subject of another report.

Thus, our investigations justify the conclusion that there is a relatively high prevalence of chronic functional psychoses in Ireland in the area served by the Three County Psychiatric Case Register. This may have come about through:

1. a high incidence of schizophrenia in the past and also currently;
2. a poor prognosis and outcome for the condition because of (*a*) an inherently unfavourable natural history or (*b*) poor treatment.

The question of a relatively high incidence currently has been investigated through our participation in the WHO study (1984) 'Determinants of outcome of severe mental disorders'. This consists of a core study which is concerned with establishing the incidence of the condition in the various participating centres. Our preliminary results do not indicate that a raised incidence exists in the three counties investigated in the study.

The question of a high incidence in the past as an explanation has gained some support from a recent study undertaken by us jointly with service and visiting personnel in one of our three counties. This study involves the intensive investigation of a geographical area within the county known to the local service providers as being a high mental illness pocket. The population of the area was just under 3000. The area was studied during a six-monthly period and all existing and arising cases of psychoses during this time were identified from the case register and by the key informant method. Each case was individually examined and diagnoses were made by either the resident or visiting psychiatrist in accordance with DSM-III. 38 persons were diagnosed as suffering from schizophrenia (ICD 295 and schizoaffective disorder, 295.7). A few other persons with schizophrenic symptoms were excluded from the study either because of coexisting organic disorders or because of an onset aged over 45. The rate of schizophrenia based on 38 active cases works out as 1.3% (Torrey *et al.*, 1984). This is higher than any previously recorded prevalence figure, the nearest being 0.9% which comes from Böök's Northern Sweden study, analysed in a fashion comparable to our own data (Böök, 1953).

Thus it is inescapable that the high schizophrenia prevalence in Ireland may well be the consequence of a raised incidence in the past. That the figures given are not the consequence of artefactual distortions such as those brought about by migration was excluded in the following fashion. The mean age of the group of 36 prevalence patients was 56 years. The population of the area under consideration at that time was 4800 (the population has fallen by 1800 persons since 1926). Making appropriate allowance for the population differential and assuming that none of those who out-migrated became ill the schizophrenia prevalence rate of this population drops to 7.5 per 1000. The corrected figure although just lower than Böök's still remains extremely high.

If the raised past incidence be contrasted with the apparently unremarkable present incidence then we are led to conclude that a most interesting change in schizophrenia incidence has occurred within the last half century in this area. The consequences of this change in incidence are of enormous scientific interest and we hope to investigate them further.

Unfavourable outcome

The other possibility of a relatively unfavourable outcome for Irish schizophrenia cases is being investigated through our participation in the 'Disability sub-study' of the WHO (1984) multicentre collaborative study on 'Determinants of outcome of severe mental disorders'. Here three annual groups of incidence schizophrenia cases have been gathered by the case register and each has been followed through for a number of years to assess the rate of disability and impairment development over the period of study. This is being done by the use of standardized instruments such as the Disability Assessment Schedule and the Impairments Rating Scale. It will thus be possible to compare the rate of disability and impairment development in the Irish groups compared with the others. This should go some way to answering the question whether the rate of deterioration progression is greater in the Irish group than in the others. At the same time an attempt is being made to determine the effect of various socio-cultural influences on deterioration rate.

Pilot study areas

The case register is also being used to follow the outcome of patients already in care and patients entering care during a defined period in a WHO collaborative study taking place in 21 pilot study areas throughout the European region (WHO, 1984).

Further uses to which it is hoped the case register will be put will be another study in the area of cost-effectiveness of psychiatric services. Here the project will make a comparison between the St Loman's service, which uses a policy of short hospitalization and intensive community care, compared with one of the three counties where long hospitalization and dependence on institutional care rather than community alternatives has been the predominant policy.

As the case register provides extensive family data it is also being used as the basic tool for a family study of the human leukocytic antigen (HLA) constitution of affected schizophrenic persons and their first and second degree relatives (preliminary data indicate that 60% of schizophrenic individuals have affected first degree relatives). This study is of particular interest because of the large family size in Ireland not now seen elsewhere in western Europe.

Summary

This paper has tried to give some indication of the nature of psychiatric case registers, their disposition in Europe and has illustrated the uses to which they can be put in following patients over long periods of time and thus evaluating their outcome. Administrative as well as the scientific aspects of chronic functional psychoses can thus be studied from a base or sample frame previously unavailable.

References

Baldwin, J. A. (1974). The Oxford Register. In *Proceedings of the Conference on Psychiatric Case Registers at the University of Aberdeen March* 1973. Statistical and Research Report Series No. 7. Department of Health and Social Security. London: Her Majesty's Stationery Office.

Baldwin, J. A., Innes, G., Millar, W. M., Sharp, G. & Dorricott, N. (1965). A psychiatric case register in north-east Scotland. *British Journal of Preventive and Social Medicine*, **19**, 38–42.

Böök, J. A. (1953). A genetic and neuropsychiatric investigation of a north Swedish population, with special regard to schizophrenia and mental deficiency. *Acta Genetica*, **4**, 1–100, 133–9, 345–414.

Council of Europe, European Committee on Legal Co-operation (CDCJ) (1982). *Protection of Personal Data used for Scientific Research and Statistics*. Strasbourg: Council of Europe.

Department of Health and Social Security (1971). *The Nottingham Psychiatric Case Register Findings* 1962 *to* 1969. Statistical Report Series No. 13. London: Her Majesty's Stationery Office.

Dupont, A., Videbech, T. & Weeke, A. (1974). A cumulative national psychiatric case register: its structure and application. *Acta Psychiatrica Scandinavica*, **50**, 161–73.

Fryers, T. & Wooff, K. (1974). The Salford Register. In *Proceedings of the Conference on Psychiatric Case Registers at the University of Aberdeen March 1973*. Statistical and Research Report Series No. 7. Department of Health and Social Security. London: Her Majesty's Stationery Office.

Giel, R. & ten Horn, G. H. M. M. (1982). Patterns of mental health care in a Dutch register area. *Social Psychiatry*, **17**, 117–23.

Grad de Alarcon, J. & Nelson, B. (1974). The Southampton Register. In *Proceedings of the Conference on Psychiatric Case Registers at the University of Aberdeen March 1973*. Statistical and Research Report Series No. 7. Department of Health and Social Security. London: Her Majesty's Stationery Office.

Häfner, H. & Klug, J. (1982). The impact of an expanding community mental health service on patterns of bed usage: evaluation of a four-year period of implementation. *Psychological Medicine*, **12**, 177–90.

niNuallain, M., Buckley, H., McHugh, B., O'Hare, A. & Walsh, D. (1984). Methodology for a study of mental illness in Ireland. *Irish Journal of Psychiatry*, **15**, 4–10.

Torre, E., Marinoni, A. & Allegri, G. (1982). Lomest psychiatric case register: old and new long-stay patients. *Social Psychiatry*, **17**, 125–31.

Torrey, E. F., McGuire, M., O'Hare, A., Walsh, D. & Spellman, M. P. (1984). Endemic psychosis in western Ireland. *American Journal of Psychiatry*, **141** (8), 966–70.

Walsh, D., Butler, S. & Starks, S. (1981). The St Loman's psychiatric service: an exercise in parisomy. *Irish Journal of Psychiatry*, (autumn) 9–22.

Walsh, D., O'Hare, A., Blake, B., Halpenny, J. V. & O'Brien, P. F. (1980). The treated prevalence of mental illness in the Republic of Ireland – the three county case register study. *Psychological Medicine*, **10**, 465–70.

Walsh, B. & Walsh, D. (1970). Mental illness in the Republic of Ireland – first admissions. *Journal of the Irish Medical Association*, **63** (400), 365–70.

Wing, J. K. & Fryers, T. (eds) (1976). *Statistics from the Camberwell and Salford Registers 1964–1974*. Institute of Psychiatry: London/Department of Community Medicine: University of Manchester.

World Health Organization (1984). *Mental Health Services in Pilot Study Areas*. Copenhagen: WHO, Regional Office.

Social disability and chronic mental disorder

R. GIEL, A. DEJONG, C. J. SLOOFF AND D. WIERSMA

Introduction

Chronic disability is a common feature of serious mental illness. Its relationship with psychopathology, particularly in terms of the nature and gravity of symptoms as assessed with the aid of diagnostic interviews and classified with systems like ICD-9 or DSM-III, has not yet been adequately established.

The ability to assess precisely the nature and consequences of chronic disability is becoming more urgent because of the trend towards avoiding long-term hospitalization. In a recent longitudinal investigation in Groningen, under the umbrella of the 'WHO Collaborative Study on the Assessment and Reduction of Psychiatric Disability' (Jablensky, Schwarz & Tomov, 1980) we followed a group of people over a period of 3 years. This comprised patients who, for the first time in their lives, manifested symptoms of non-affective functional psychosis (Wiersma *et al.*, 1984*b*). It appeared that those with non-remitting or frequently recurring psychosis had, on average, spent less than 40% of their time in hospital. This was, in fact, somewhat less than people with a few limited psychotic episodes. In Fig. 1, each dot represents a patient in one of the subgroups with a particular course of psychosis during the first 3 years after the onset of the illness. The solid line connects the average percentage of time spent in hospital by the various subgroups. The broken line represents the same for any type of care. To give an example, the figure shows that nine patients in the two categories with the worst course (IV^a and IV^b) spent less than 20% of the period in hospital. This could be considered a satisfactory situation, but it was also found that the course taken by their disability was anything but favourable. The development of social disability did not parallel that of symptomatology. For the same subgroups, Fig. 2 illustrates the manner in which the disability developed over 3 years. Disability was

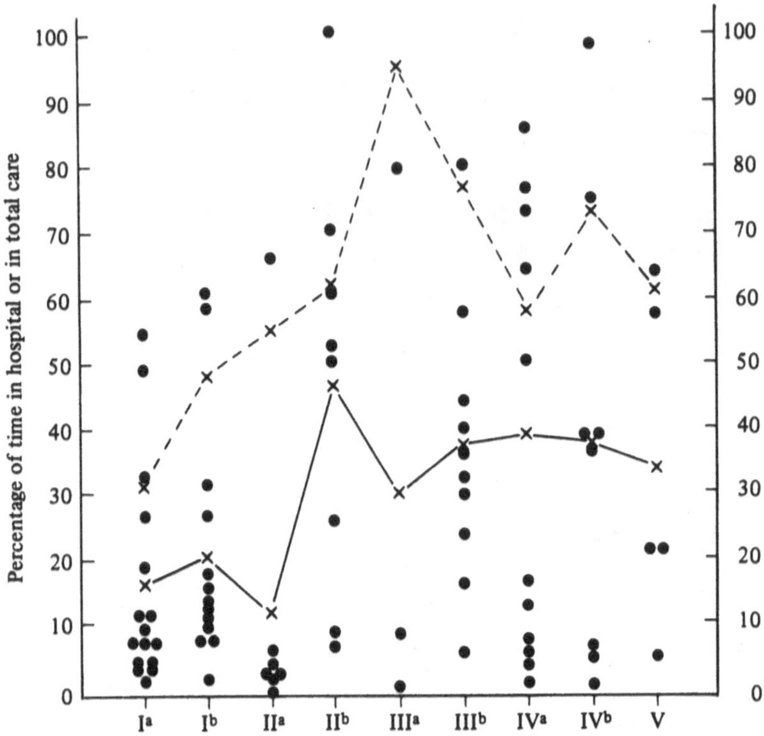

Fig. 1. Percentages of time in hospital according to the course of functional psychosis. Solid line, mean percentage of time in hospital; broken line, mean percentage of time in total care, including ambulatory care. I[a], one episode plus complete remission (n = 16); I[b], two or more episodes plus complete remission (n = 13); II[a], one episode plus neurotic syndrome (n = 8); II[b], two or more episodes plus neurotic syndrome (n = 8); III[a], one episode plus personality change (n = 3); III[b], two or more episodes plus personality change (n = 10); IV[a], chronic psychosis (n = 11); IV[b], several lengthy episodes (n = 8); V, deceased (suicide; n = 5).

measured using the Disability Assessment Schedule (Jablensky *et al.*, 1980) and counted as the sum of the scores on the individual sections. In subgroup I[b], the deterioration of functioning, despite the complete remission of symptoms after the psychotic episodes, is remarkable.

These findings stress the need for an assessment of disability independent from that of psychopathology in order to direct social rehabilitation, particularly for people suffering from chronic psychosis (though not limited to that group). Unfortunately, there is a lack of both uniform and unambiguous descriptive terminology of social disability and models of social (dys)functioning. These would be of great help to any successful study of the development of social disability and its relationship with psychopathology. In this respect, social psychiatry lags behind clinical

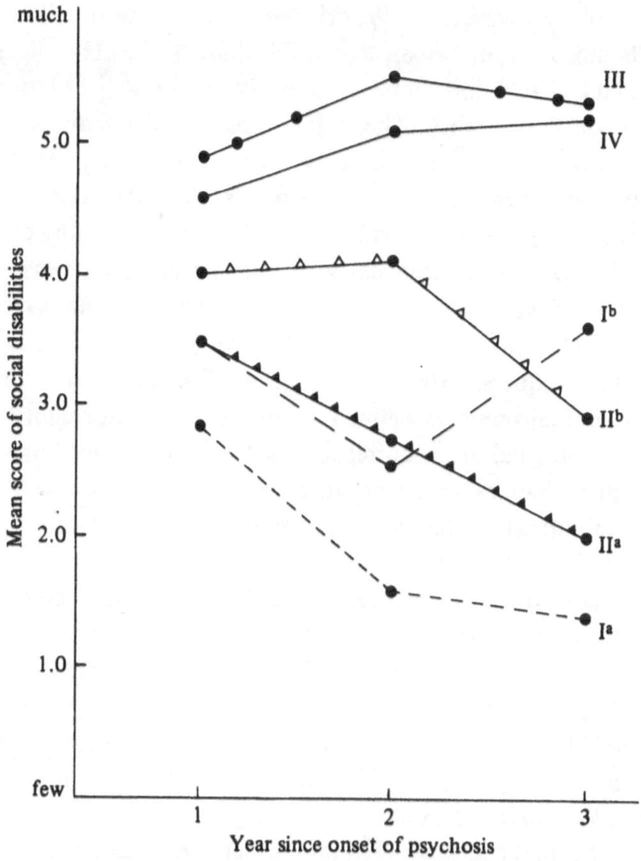

Fig. 2. The course of social disabilities according to the course of functional psychosis (excluding five suicides). III, one or more episodes plus personality change ($n = 13$); IV, (nearly) chronic psychosis ($n = 19$); I[b], two or more episodes plus complete remission; II[b], two or more episodes plus neurotic syndrome; II[a], one episode plus neurotic syndrome; I[a], one episode plus complete remission.

psychiatry, the latter having developed (for example) biochemical and psychodynamic causal models to aid in the understanding of individual mental disorders. In the case of schizophrenia, conceptualization in terms of impaired cognitive abilities, i.e. as a weakening of attention and perception processes (Venables, 1978), perhaps comes closest to a theory which could largely explain the development of social disability.

Terminology

At a symposium of the section of Epidemiology and Community Psychiatry of the World Psychiatric Association in Baltimore held in 1982, Gruenberg & Pepper (1982) attempted to clear up some of the terminological issues by defining mental illness, patient, disability and chronicity as accurately as possible. However, the World Health Organization (WHO) International Classification of Impairments, Disabilities, and Handicaps (ICIDH; see WHO, 1980) has gone furthest in defining the various concepts which underly disability. The ICIDH specifies the sequence of illness-related phenomena in the following manner: disease ↦ impairment ↦ disability ↦ handicap. In fact, this broadening of the concept of disease, including the impairments, disabilities and handicaps arising from it, is a prerequisite for the fruitful study of chronic mental illness. In practice, the term chronic refers not only to the duration of the disease in a restricted sense (aetiology, pathology and manifestation) but also to the duration of its consequences (impairments, disabilities and handicaps).

In the ICIDH, 'impairment' is defined as any loss or abnormality of psychological, physiological or anatomical structure or function. Impairments represent disturbances at the organ or system level. They can be experienced by the patient in the form of symptoms, or be observed by others as deviations.

'Disability' is defined as any restriction or lack (resulting from an impairment) of the ability to perform an activity in the manner or within the range considered normal for a human being. Disabilities may result directly from an impairment or as a consequence of a person's awareness of his impairment. The concept of disability is concerned with compound or integrated activities expected of the person as a whole, such as are represented by tasks, skills and behaviour.

Disabilities constitute the link between impairment and 'handicap'. The latter term is defined as a disadvantage for a given individual resulting from an impairment or disability, which limits or prevents fulfilment of a role that is normal (depending on age, sex, social and cultural factors) for that individual. The state of being handicapped is relative to other people, whose attitudes and responses play a key role in defining the possibilities of an individual who is disabled, for example, by attaching a stigma to the disability. The ICIDH seems to imply that disabilities should be measured by universal human standards, whereas handicaps are sociocultural phenomena.

The ICIDH represents an important step in the description and classification of diseases and their effects. However, for a variety of reasons much further research remains to be done before it can be successfully applied in psychiatry. First and foremost, it poses a number of conceptual problems, and second, just like the ICD, it fails to provide adequate operational criteria.

Perhaps one of the basic conceptual problems in the definition of impairments and disabilities concerns the delineation of mental systems (following the analogy of the organs and systems featuring in somatic medicine) as opposed to functions and activities of the whole individual. If one accepts that the relationship between the first sequence (disease or disorder) and the second (the consequences in the form of impairments, disabilities and handicaps) is a worthy subject for research, the distinction between the manifestations of pathology (symptoms) and impairments should be clarified. Unfortunately, the ICIDH already mixes the two concepts in its explanatory text. For example, depersonalization is rated as a pathological subjective experience, and therefore as a symptom. In the ICIDH it can be rated as an impairment (see 23.30 'Other psychological impairment: impairments of perception and attention'). It would also appear as a self-awareness disability, however (10.0 'Disturbance of the ability to develop or maintain a mental representation of the identity of the individual's self or body and its continuity over time').

By the same token, the conceptualization of disabilities versus handicaps also poses considerable problems. In both cases a psychiatrist would be inclined to think in terms of social role performance. In consequence it will become difficult to see how disabilities should be assessed by more universal human standards when, in judging handicaps, sociocultural norms have to be used. The ICIDH itself confused the issue when it introduced customary activities such as going out together or visiting other people, to assess family role disability. To some extent, the handicaps section of the ICIDH is a summary of the impairment and disability section.

In our view the ICIDH is a useful first step towards the classification of the consequences of chronic mental illness and, because of this, should be given priority as an area of research. Studies should include scrutiny of concepts, definition of operational criteria for its classes once the concepts have been clarified, and finally its reliability and validity should be tested on extensively documented cases of various types of mental disorder by professionals from different disciplines.

Models of social disability

In the Netherlands, one out of every four people labelled as medically unfit for employment in 1980 under the terms of disability legislation was qualified as such on psychiatric grounds (de Jong *et al.*, 1983). In 1970 this reason applied to only one in seven or eight disability cases. It is unlikely that during the past decade morbidity changed dramatically, nor is there any indication that treatment of mental disorders has deteriorated to such a degree as to explain this worsening situation, which reflects not only a relative but also an absolute increase in psychiatric disability. It may be that changes in the definition of disability are involved here.

Apparently, the straightforward model of the ICIDH depicting the sequence from disease to disability is too simple. Slater *et al.* (1980) suggested a complex of factors which contributed to the qualification of disability: a patient's perception of himself, the restrictions in his performance which he is likely to report, evaluation of the patient's performance by key figures in his environment, evaluation by the medical profession (which is not only based on dysfunctions but also on diagnosis and prognosis), legal criteria, and normative responses from the community. It should be clear that the majority of these factors could also determine the permanence of disability, even in the case of a favourable psychopathological outcome. By long-term follow-up studies of schizophrenia – generally thought to contribute heavily to serious mental handicap – Gross & Huber (1973) and Ciompi & Müller (1976) showed that 49–58% of their cases had a favourable outcome from the psychopathological viewpoint. Obviously, a model of social disability should not just include a complex of factors contributing to its emergence and continuation, but also allow the study of its progression and regression. In this respect Cooper's (1980) proposal for a taxonomic hierarchy (see the appendix to this chapter) might be helpful. It ranks disability in the context of:

Rank 8 Origins: race, nation, tribe, cultural groups;

Rank 7 Affiliation: profession, union, minor religious groups;

Rank 6 Groups: small group roles, such as in the family and at work;

Rank 5 Dyadic: relationships and roles;

Rank 4 Control: individual response to and control of immediate environment;

Rank 3 Awareness: psychological function and behaviour sequence;

Rank 2 Homeostasis: physiological homeostasis and simple movements;

Rank 1 Anatomy: the body with its organs.

While Rank 3 seems to refer to the level of impairments in the ICIDH, Ranks 4–8 relate to the levels of social disabilities and handicaps. It should be added that Cooper included more details than given here. The hierarchy will need much further work, however, both with regard to the description of the ranks and their various classes of behaviour and to the criteria for classification. Progression and regression of disability can be monitored by the manner of expansion or retraction from one rank or level of dysfunctioning to another, or as it expands within a particular rank.

Conclusion

The development of models of social disability requires further elaboration of Cooper's taxonomic hierarchy and of the theoretical framework of the ICIDH.

In our study we tried to reproduce a hierarchy of social disability with the results of the Disability Assessment Schedule. We succeeded in constructing a one-dimensional scale on the basis of seven disability items, ranging from work role, heterosexual role, social contacts, general interest, leisure time activities and participation in the household, to self-care. This sequence appears to correspond to Cooper's ranks 7, 6, 5 and 4 to some extent. The results of our follow-up of non-affective functionally psychotic patients suggested a progression of social disability from ranks 7 to 4 as the psychopathological condition becomes more severe, also over time (Wiersma *et al.*, 1983, 1984*a*). We have arrived at the following hypotheses which, in our view, deserve to be tested:

1. Social disability tends to develop in a hierarchical fashion, depending on the severity of psychopathology.
2. The course taken by social disability is relatively independent of the course of psychopathology.
3. Social disability is not specifically related to diagnosis.
4. A patient's environmental circumstances are of greater importance to progression or regression of social disability than his personal characteristics.

It is a prerequisite, however, to undertake longitudinal research groups of patients with narrowly specified and symptomatically homogeneous psychiatric conditions, and to include patients from the onset of disease. Therefore our efforts are, at present, aimed at the development of a system of classifying psychological impairments and social disabilities, and at testing its validity, reliability and applicability with regard to groups of psychiatric and other patients.

APPENDIX

Rank 8: Origins: Race, nation, tribe, cultural groups

Rank 7: Affiliation: Profession, union, minor religious groups

Rank 6: Groups: Small group roles

Family	*Domestic*	*Social*
Father	Breadwinner	Leisure groups
Mother	Housekeeper	Neighbourhood groups
Son, daughter		

Group skills	*Work*
Group manners	Task group roles
Travel and casual groups	Work/social roles

Rank 5: Dyadic: Relationships and roles

Personal	*Social skills*	*Social status*
Marital	Verbal	Hierarchical position behaviour
Parental	Non-verbal	
Sibling	Dyadic manners	
Sexual	Coping with change in relationships	
Mimetic learning		

Supportive
Provider
Career

Rank 4: Control: Individual response to and control of immediate environment

Personal comfort	*Intellect and information*
Social procedures for eating, excreting washing dressing handling money	Read, write, draw Make decisions, cope with change Operant learning

Emotional control	*Physical activity*
Control of affective responses	Use of tools to manipulate environment
Fight, flight and sex response	Work activity sequences

Rank 3: Awareness: Psychological function and behaviour sequence

Alimentary	*Arousal*
Mechanisms for drinking eating excretion	Orientation, concentration, attention Memory, learning Conditioned learning

	Affect and sensorium Normal affect and perception Special senses functions (speech, vision, hearing, etc.)	*Movement sequence* Walk, jump, run Push, grip, lift
Rank 2:	Homeostasis: Physiological homeostasis and simple movements	
	Physiological systems Cardiovascular, renal Respiratory Hormonal, blood, etc.	*CNS* Reflex responses Reflex learning
	Simple movements Simple individual muscle and joint movements	
Rank 1:	Anatomy: The body Intact organs Intact CNS	Intact joints and limbs

From: Cooper, J. E. (1980).

References

Ciompi, L. & Müller, C. (1976). *Lebensweg und Alter der Schizophrenen*. Berlin: Springer Verlag.

Cooper, J. E. (1980). The description and classification of social disability by means of a taxonomic hierarchy. In *Epidemiological Research as Basis for the Organization of Extramural Psychiatry, Acta Psychiatrica Scandinavica*, Suppl. 285, **62**, 140–6.

Gross, G. & Huber, G. (1973). Zur Prognose der Schizophrenien. *Psychiatria Clinica*, **6**, 1–16.

Gruenberg, E. M. & Pepper, B. (1982). Definition of I. Mental illness, II. Patient, III. Disability and IV. Chronic. Paper presented during the World Psychiatric Association Conference of the Chronically Mentally Ill, An International Perspective. Baltimore: John Hopkins University.

Jablensky, A., Schwarz, R. & Tomov, T. (1980). WHO Collaborative Study on impairments and disabilities associated with schizophrenic disorders. A preliminary communication: objectives and methods. *Acta Psychiatrica Scandinavica*, Suppl. 285.

Jong, A. de, Giel, R., Slooff, C. J. & Wiersma, D. (1983). Sociale beperkingen ten gevolge van funktionele psychosen. I. Een ontwerp voor een model voor de ontwikkeling van sociale beperkingen. *Tijdschrift voor Sociale Gezondheidszorg*, **61**, 78–85.

Slater, S. B., Vulmanovic, C., Macukanovic, P., Prvulovic, T. & Cutler, J. L. (1980). The definition and measurement of disability. *Social Science and Medicine*, **8**, 305–8.

Venables, P. H. (1978). Cognitive Disorder. In *Schizophrenia: Towards a New Synthesis*, ed. J. K. Wing. London: Academic Press.

Wiersma, D., Jong, A. de, Giel, R. & Slooff, C. J. (1983). Sociale beperkingen tengevolge van funktionele psychosen. II. Enkele bevindingen betreffende het model voor de ontwikkeling van sociale beperkingen. *Tijdschrift voor Sociale Gezondheidszorg*, **61**, 168–74.

Wiersma, D., Giel, R., Jong, A. de, Slooff, C. J. (1984*a*). Measuring social disability in schizophrenic patients. Paper presented during the World Psychiatric Association Conference of the Chronically Mentally Ill. An International Perspective. Baltimore: John Hopkins University.

Wiersma, D., Giel, R., Jong, A. de & Slooff, C. J. (1984*b*) Chroniciteit bij functionele psychosen. *Tijdschrift voor psychiatrie*, **6**, no. 6.

World Health Organization (1980). *International Classification of Impairments, Disabilities and Handicaps*. Geneva: WHO.

The neglect of the patient with chronic functional psychosis: the need for further research

R. G. PRIEST, P. RAPTOPOULOS AND
M. L. CHAN

(Paper read by R.G.P.)

Introduction

It is understandable that throughout medicine the treatment of acute disorders has a greater emotional appeal than the management of long-term disability. Psychiatrists in particular should be able to understand the strong motivational bias that ensures that attention is paid to patients in crisis and with emergencies. It is the chronic patient who gets neglected.

The hospital system is geared to the needs of acute disorders. As the patients are discharged into the community so the links with their specialists become more tenuous. Where general practitioners are well trained, they can take over the patients' care, but this transfer is in itself fraught with danger. Although many hospital specialists (including myself) have undertaken an early apprenticeship in general practice, it is unusual for the hospital specialist to become a full-time family doctor at a mature stage. Professor Francis Kellerman, a specialist in diseases of the chest, did just that. He has written about his experiences recently (Kellerman, 1983) and I should like to quote his comments about patients with psychiatric disorders:

> The most frustrating surprise concerned the mentally ill. There is no doubt that when the NHS [National Health Service] was introduced a drastic reform of the care and treatment of the mentally ill was long overdue, and in quick succession a number of mental health acts were passed, putting many wrongs right – and just as many rights wrong.
>
> Before the recent mental health acts, the mentally ill were cared for in mental homes [mental hospitals].
>
> Today, with the help of a combination of powerful psychotropic drugs, they are 'cured' in the hospital and then go home – often against the better judgement of the consultant in charge.

> At home, because of non-compliance, or a number of other factors, they relapse. This may take weeks, months or years, but in my experience, in the more severe forms of psychoses, the relapsing rate is nearly 100 per cent.

It is not surprising that a large number of patients fall out of the care network. Chronic psychiatric subjects roam the streets, dressed in shabby clothes, rummaging in dustbins and occasionally shouting out loud to nobody in particular.

Anderson (1923) classified homeless men into three types. Firstly there are the itinerant workers – the hobos. Secondly there are the itinerant non-workers – the tramps. Thirdly there are the non-itinerant non-workers – the bums. In France the approximate equivalents are the *errants*, the *vagabonds* and the *clochards*. It has been stated (Ey, 1957) that 'the problem of the *clochard* is not essentially psychiatric and it would be ridiculous to think that *clochards* are all patients, neurotics or psychotics'. But would it? I shall come back to this point.

It is increasingly recognized that the degrading process of institutionalization can take place in the community as well as in the mental hospital. Are there circumstances in which it would be preferable to be a patient in a long-stay ward in a large psychiatric hospital rather than have the freedom to live a less ordered life?

The current pattern of care

Although I have spent much of my life working in large psychiatric hospitals, my current clinical base is a 58-bed psychiatric unit in a district general hospital (DGH). Typically a psychotic patient is admitted as an emergency with suicidal feelings, severe depression or bizarre behaviour, or often all of these. Our unit deals with all adult patients from a defined catchment area who need hospitalization for functional mental illness. We took this catchment area over from the distant large mental hospital that previously served it.

In many ways our wards resemble in their function the admission wards of a mental hospital. It is the policy of the British Department of Health and Social Security (DHSS) to close down large mental hospitals and provide more DGH psychiatric units, of a size of 60–120 beds, at roughly 60 beds to 100000 members of the population.

In recent years, the focus of treatment of the mentally ill has been changing from compulsory treatment in the asylum (Jones, 1972) to care based on open-door hospital units, day-hospitals, out-patient clinics (on the hospital side) linked with day centres, hostels, group homes and other sheltered community facilities (on the part of the social service departments).

The Government paper *Better Services for the Mentally Ill* (DHSS, 1975*a*) paints a picture of a parallel system of care, the new existing alongside the old, with an ideal service unlikely 'within even a twenty-five year planning horizon' (p. iii).

The district psychiatric units are not intended to refer their chronic and difficult cases to the local mental hospital. No-one knows at present how fast long-stay patients will accumulate in the new units and what proportion of the beds will remain for the acute patients.

The 58-bed psychiatric unit at St Mary's Hospital, London W9 took on catchment area responsibility in 1977. We have analysed the data for the first two years' admissions (Priest, Raptopoulos & Chan, 1979). I suppose that we had expected a unimodal distribution of length of stay and an average length of stay of about 6–8 weeks. The distribution that we found is displayed on the accompanying histogram (see Appendix 1 to this chapter). The commonest duration of stay is up to 1 week with subsequent frequencies falling away week by week. It struck me that this picture was very similar to an exponential decay curve and this interpretation was supported by curve fitting (method of least squares). There was a correlation co-efficient of 0.87 with the exponential equation

$$y = ae^{-bx} \; (y = a\exp(-bx))$$

where $a = 48.5$

and $b = 0.11$.

The areas in which the frequencies exceeded the theoretical distribution were in the patients staying 1 week or less and those staying over 26 weeks. Often patients are discharged or take their own discharge on the day of admission or soon afterwards and these are possibly inappropriate admissions in the first place. Those staying over 26 weeks may include patients whose stay in hospital is no longer necessary but for whom there is no adequate provision of sheltered accommodation in the community. If lengths of stay of over 26 weeks are ignored a correlation co-efficient of 0.93 is obtained.

It will be interesting to see if others can confirm these findings since, if the theoretical distribution is a good approximation, then much more powerful forecasts could be made. Preliminary investigations suggest that the national data are also exponential in nature but with different parameters. It is somewhat humbling to find that the behaviour of the population follows a simple mathematical law although linear changes in population have been described earlier (Tooth & Brooke, 1961; Priest, 1972*b*).

Although the number of psychiatric beds has fallen steadily (DHSS, 1975*b*), both out-patient attendances and the number of admissions have been rising. It is likely that the new pattern of care will speed up this process. Patients with acute illnesses are likely to seek treatment in general hospital units in higher numbers than would have contemplated going to the mental hospital. In some cases admission may be inappropriate (despite the demands of the patient) but in others the reasons for admission could be more compelling. It is a common gibe that there are more mentally ill outside hospital than in; for every one person in a psychiatric ward there may be ten or so equally disturbed in the community (Crisp & Priest, 1971). Apart from increased numbers of referrals by general practitioners, the DGH units are likely to uncover cross-referrals from other hospital physicians.

It is hoped that in the new units there will be less tendency for patients with chronic illness involving impaired social function to continue to use hospital beds when they could better be using sheltered care in the community. Those working in mental hospitals are familiar with patients who have lingered from inertia, are now comfortable in the artificial environment and who fear the cold winds that blow outside. It would certainly seem that this is less likely to happen in the smaller district units, so the problems of institutionalization (Wing & Brown, 1970) should be less, assuming that community care facilities are available.

Another foreseeable development is the community care of clients who are less remediable than those currently attending day centres and living in hostels. So far, day centres have tended to prefer clients for whom they could see some hope of rehabilitation. Hostels have selected preferentially those that were able to hold down a job. We have yet to detect the full consequences of managing out of hospital those who will continue to need sheltered housing and sheltered occupation for an indefinite period.

There are various problems with this plan. The hostels and sheltered workshops are to be provided by the Local Authorities (i.e. the city governing councils, financed particularly by property taxes) who have a different set of priorities to the national, central Government (financed particularly by income tax). The difference in priorities means that the hostels and sheltered workshops do not always match the numbers of hospital beds, and patients are discharged from hospital with no suitable facilities in the community to welcome them.

Recommendation

The scientific intervention required here is at the stage of data collection and observation, using descriptive statistics rather than inferential statistics.

We require a quantified flow chart. Out of each 100 admissions, how many will require hostel accommodation on discharge, how many group homes, how many day centre facilities, how many sheltered workshops? My colleague Dr Paul Raptopoulos and I have designed a coding sheet that can be used to record such data (see Appendix 2 to this chapter) and we have already obtained some information on its reliability (P. Raptopoulos, R. G. Priest & C. Syme, unpublished). With the knowledge of the numbers involved, we can begin to plan rationally for the provision of the required facilities.

The chronic relapsing patient

There are some misconceptions about the operation of the British National Health Service (NHS). In the USA there are widespread misgivings about what they refer to as 'socialized medicine' and in particular it is commonly believed there that the British patient has no choice in his general practitioner (GP) but is assigned by the authorities to a particular doctor. This is not true (except in special circumstances, such as with an especially difficult patient!).

However there is a degree of rigidity in the system. In general it is not possible for a patient to arrange to see a psychiatrist of his choice under the NHS. He needs to have a letter of referral from his own family doctor. The GP in turn is limited by the notion of the 'catchment area' – each psychiatric unit serves a defined geographical area and is likely to refuse to accept patients from elsewhere.

Earlier (in the introduction) I illustrated some of the problems that can arise with the chronic relapsing patient when the roles of the GP and the psychiatrist conflict. Add to this the propensity of such patients to wander from one area to another, and you can see that it is all too easy for a patient to fall out of care. For lack of encouragement he stops taking his medication, and is admitted once more in relapse, possibly to a new hospital and a new psychiatric team who do not have the advantage of previous acquaintance with him.

What is the scale of this problem? At present we do not know. To complement the flow data, the collection of which was recommended above, what is needed here is a cross-sectional approach in which, on a given date, the number of patients in a given area are ascertained at various levels:

1. those in the community but not being treated by their GPs,
2. those being treated by GPs alone,
3. those attending psychiatric out-patients,
4. those attending psychiatric day-hospitals,
5. those who are in-patients in psychiatric units.

To ensure that a comparison can be made of their degree of psychopathology, the same psychometric tests should be administered to samples of each of these five levels.

Psychometric tests

Much has been done in recent years to find objective measures of mental status using psychometric techniques. A measure (e.g. a questionnaire) will be regarded as objective when it is standardized, when there are normative data for it, and when it has a known reliability and validity. I have had some experience in the use of these techniques (Priest, 1969*a*, 1970, 1971*a*, 1971*b*, 1972*a*, 1972*b*, 1976*a*, 1976*b*), and I have been able to confirm their suitability in surveys in a variety of settings including a psychiatric hospital (Priest, Tarighati & Shariatmadari, 1969; Priest, Shariatmadari & Tarighati, 1973), general hospital units (Priest, 1971*b*, 1972*b*, 1976*b*; Priest & Netter, 1975), subjects in the general population who were registered with a general practitioner though not necessarily attending him (Crisp & Priest, 1971; Priest & Crisp, 1973) and those in the community thought to be at high risk (Priest, 1969*a*, 1970, 1971*a*, 1976*a*).

In particular I have been interested in the interaction of psychiatric morbidity (as measured on these instruments, as well as clinically) with social problems (e.g. homelessness and unwanted pregnancy) and the ways in which those presenting to the mental health services differ from those who remain untreated in the community despite having similar social problems (Priest, 1976*a*) or similar symptoms (Crisp & Priest, 1971).

Using these psychometric tools, patients may be categorized in a number of ways. Firstly morbidity may be assessed by judging the general level of emotional distress. This is done in the Personal Illness and Personal Disturbance scales of the Symptom-Sign Inventory (SSI, Foulds, 1965; Foulds & Hope, 1968; Priest *et al.*, 1973; Priest, 1971*a*, 1971*b*, 1972*b*, 1976*a*) or the more recent states of Anxiety and Depression (sAD) scale from the Delusions-Symptoms-States Inventory (DSSI) of Foulds & Bedford (A. Bedford, personal communication; Foulds & Bedford, 1975; Foulds, Bedford & Csapo, 1975). The General Health Questionnaire

(GHQ) is a device of this sort which has proved its value as a survey instrument in general practice and in a community based psychiatric service (Goldberg, 1972; Sims & Salmons, 1975).

Alternatively, psychometric tests are available that allocate the patient to a specific clinical diagnosis, or that at least provide a profile along a series of diagnostic alternatives. In this group we have the full 80-item SSI (Foulds, 1965; Foulds & Hope, 1968; Priest, 1971*a*, 1976*a*) which is completed by the observer, the development of this known as the DSSI which is completed by the subject (Foulds & Bedford, 1975; Foulds *et al.*, 1975), or the Middlesex Hospital Questionnaire which is confined to neurotic, as opposed to psychotic, diagnoses (Crisp & Priest, 1971; Priest & Crisp, 1973). A special type of observer-rated diagnostic inventory is the standardized clinical interview, e.g. the Present State Examination (Wing, Cooper & Sartorius, 1974; Priest, 1975).

Both observer ratings and self ratings have their merits. Guy, Gross & Dennis (1967) have discussed the influence of the observer on assessment results. To avoid observer bias, especially when the rater is aware of the hypothesis under test, there is something to be said for self-rating scales.

Problems of identifying the chronic psychotic patient

Self-rating scales pose problems when dealing with psychotic patients. The problem of the validity of their answers is considered elsewhere (Priest, 1969*b*). Perhaps a more serious problem is that of compliance. Not all patients are able or prepared to complete a questionnaire containing a systematic enquiry about their symptoms.

There is a further, even more serious, difficulty. The identification of a patient with functional mental illness by symptom-rating scales relies heavily (whether explicitly or not) on the presence of neurotic symptoms, in particular anxiety and depressive symptoms. Foulds (1965) and his colleagues found that whereas neurotic patients have neurotic symptoms, psychotic patients have psychotic symptoms but also *just as many neurotic symptoms as do the neurotic patients themselves*. That this fact had not been earlier recognized was attributed by Foulds to what he called the 'King Lear' principle. Shakespeare makes his main character affirm that

> where the greater malady is fix'd,
> The lesser is scarce felt.
> (King Lear, Act III, Scene IV).

I think that this is true in a metaphorical rather than a literal sense, but further research has provided ample confirmation of Foulds' findings.

The upshot is that when brief scales are derived empirically from larger questionnaires, it is especially the anxiety and depressive symptoms that are good at detecting mental illness, no matter whether the illness is a neuroses or a psychosis. This certainly holds true when we are considering acute psychoses. With chronic psychoses the affective symptoms become less prominent (Priest *et al.*, 1973).

Among chronic schizophrenics, although these symptoms are still more prevalent than in the general population, only about 50% of patients exhibit the pathological levels that would be detected by symptom questionnaires. We have to develop other measures to identify chronic psychoses in surveys. It may be that self-rating questionnaires could be developed for this purpose. Modification of existing measures to include some special observer ratings is also a possibility. Dr Joan Gomez and I noticed (Gomez & Priest, 1976), when using Foulds' SSI in a long stay ward, that as well as producing the yes–no responses required for the coding according to the manual, certain other responses by the patient were also very informative.

One chronic schizophrenic patient, when asked the routine question (designed to elicit grandiose ideas) 'Have you an important mission to carry out?' suddenly sat rigidly upright then (grimacing) thumped on the table several times, then relaxed and said 'no!'. Essentially, we found that to 10 of the 80 SSI questions especially, whether or not we obtained a 'yes' response, we would get behaviour that was bizarre, thought disorder, a flow of paranoid ideas or some other indication of the underlying psychosis. Whereas in the ordinary interview the patient might fail to demonstrate overtly psychotic behaviour, the administration of these questions would elicit the production of delusional or other psychotic material.

Recommendation

A study should be performed at one point in time to identify, in a geographical area, the number of psychotic patients present at five levels:

1. those in the community but not being treated by their GPs,
2. those being treated by GPs alone,
3. those attending psychiatric out-patients,
4. those attending psychiatric day hospitals,
5. those who are in-patients in psychiatric units.

Special attention should be paid to tests that are based not just on neurotic symptoms but also on psychotic symptoms (e.g. the DSSI), general psychopathology (e.g. the Hostility and Direction of Hostility Questionnaire – HDHQ) or on direct observation of abnormal responses (Gomez & Priest, 1976).

Homeless persons

20 years ago, 30000 down-and-outs, vagabonds, tramps and other unfortunates were identified in Great Britain in the government publication *Homeless Single Persons* (HMSO, 1966). There may be even more now. The vast majority live in common lodging houses, referred to in England as 'doss-houses' and in the USA as 'flop-houses' or more formally as 'Skid-row hotels'.

I became interested in the prevalence of psychiatric disorder in this population. There were hints from epidemiological research in general that the rates might be high (Priest, 1978). Mental illness is more common in the lowest social class and in the centres of cities, which is where the lodging-houses are situated.

However there have been widely differing estimates of the prevalence of psychiatric disorder in homeless men. In the USA they are usually regarded as alcoholics. Psychiatrists from western Europe tend to think of them as chronic schizophrenics. George Orwell, who led this way of life himself (see *Down and Out in Paris and London*, or *The Road to Wigan Pier*), seemed to regard them as normal: if they had psychological problems they would be cured by getting a steady job. So what are they like – all alcoholic, all schizophrenic, all normal? I decided to carry out a systematic psychiatric study on a sample from the lodging-houses of Edinburgh (Priest, 1971*a*).

What I found was that the majority of the subjects were psychiatrically abnormal, and that the commonest diagnosis (in about a third) was overt schizophrenia. Alcoholism affected a substantial but smaller number. The results of special psychometric tests (Foulds' Symptom-Sign Inventory and the Brief Paired Associate Learning test, Priest *et al.*, 1969) were consistent with those obtained by clinical assessment.

I repeated the study in Chicago. There, alcoholism was the commonest diagnosis (in 40%), with schizophrenia coming second (Priest, 1978).

I compared the Edinburgh random sample with those patients presenting themselves to Edinburgh health services for psychiatric problems (the 'clinical series'). There were significant differences (Priest, 1976*a*). Alcoholism was rather more often diagnosed in the clinical series, and personality disorder much more often. Schizophrenia tended to be found more in the representative sample.

The schizophrenics that I had found in the representative sample rarely gave a history of mental hospital admission. It seemed that they were seeking an anonymous, unobtrusive niche in this pseudo-society, rarely talking to each other, and adopting this way of life as a preferred alternative to orthodox medical treatment.

Recommendation
I do not believe that these chronic, florid schizophrenics and other chronic psychotics discovered in random surveys should be forcibly treated against their will. However I think that it would be worthwhile trying the effect of 'shop-front' facilities in Skid-Row areas in which services were provided that they could make use of if they wished (e.g. optional extras over and above those normally supplied by the welfare state) with the goal of enticing them as voluntary patients into psychiatric treatment.

Neglected patients in mental hospitals

Some patients thrive on neglect. In my view the stimulation of interpersonal relationships is a threat which can precipitate schizophrenic breakdown (Priest & Steinert, 1977). Just as schizophrenics in the community may seek out the anonymity of the lodging-house cubicle, so some patients find greater relief in the undemanding atmosphere of a long-stay ward in a mental hospital. I have found that such patients will fiercely resist discharge. If the staff insist on returning them to the community, the relapse rate is high. By contrast, a patient whose illness remits while he is in the long-stay ward may be delighted to return to a normal life outside the hospital. Just as the disability of chronic schizophrenia may be confused with the effects of institutionalization, so the desire of a patient to remain inconspicuously in a mental hospital may be confused with neglect.

In the UK it is assumed that the large psychiatric hospitals, which have already reduced their numbers of beds substantially, will finally disappear. In their place will be psychiatric beds in the DGH backed up with community facilities. However, although progress is being made along these lines, it is proceeding slowly. The vast majority of psychiatric in-patients are still in mental hospitals rather than general hospitals. The first mental hospital has yet to close.

Will they all close? Will any close? I suspect that though the answer to the second question is yes (and fairly soon) the answer to the first is no (or at least not in my lifetime).

Recommendation
The place of the large mental hospital in psychiatric care should be re-examined. The possibility should be explored whether, even after their function as admission hospitals for a catchment area has ended, they could serve as specialist regional units. Special centres could be based there, for instance units for non-geriatric patients with organic brain disease,

alcoholism and drug dependence units, adolescent units, and medium-secure units.

The concept of the 'hospital hostel' should be explored. That is to say a high-dependency hostel, for chronic and disabled patients, situated in the community but close to the DGH psychiatric unit. This is, in essence, a case of transplanting the 'chronic ward' into the catchment area from which the patients originally came. Careful monitoring should assess whether the quality of life is better for patients there than in the 'back ward' of a mental hospital. A controlled trial of the two alternative environments is feasible.

Meanwhile, a schedule of desirable standards of care in long-stay wards should be prepared and agreed internationally.

Summary

Leaving hospital with nowhere to go

In recent years the focus of treatment of the mentally ill has been changing from compulsory treatment in the asylum (Jones, 1972) to care based on open-door hospital units, day-hospitals, out-patient clinics (on the hospital side) linked with day centres, hostels, group homes and other sheltered community facilities (on the part of the social services departments).

There are various problems with this plan. The hostels and sheltered workshops are to be provided by the Local Authorities (i.e. the city governing councils, financed particularly by property taxes) who have a different set of priorities from the national, central Government (financed particularly by income tax). The difference in priorities means that the hostels and sheltered workshops do not always match the numbers of hospital beds, and patients are discharged from hospital with no suitable facilities in the community to welcome them.

We require a quantified flow chart. Out of each 100 admissions, how many will require hostel accommodation on discharge, how many group homes, how many day centre facilities, how many sheltered workshops?

The scientific intervention required here is at the stage of data collection and observation, using descriptive rather than inferential statistics.

The chronic relapsing patient

This chapter illustrates some of the problems that can arise with the chronic relapsing patient when the roles of the GP and the psychiatrist conflict. Add to this the propensity of such patients to wander from one area to another, and it can be seen that it is easy for a patient to fall out of care. For lack of encouragement he stops taking his medication, and is admitted once more in relapse, possibly to a new hospital and a new psychiatric team who do not have the advantage of previous acquaintance with him.

What is the scale of this problem? At present we do not know. To complement the flow data, the collection of which was recommended above, what is needed here is a cross-sectional approach in which, on a given date the number of patients in a given area are ascertained at various levels:

1. those in the community but not being treated by their GPs,
2. those being treated by GPs alone,
3. those attending psychiatric out-patients,
4. those attending psychiatric day-hospitals,
5. those who are in-patients in psychiatric units.

To ensure that a comparison can be made of their degree of psychopathology, the same psychometric tests should be administered to samples of each of these five levels.

Skid Row

Surveys of 'Skid Row' populations have shown that the majority are psychiatrically abnormal, and that the commonest diagnosis is often overt schizophrenia.

The schizophrenics rarely have a history of mental hospital admission. It seems that they are seeking an anonymous, unobtrusive niche in this pseudo-society, rarely talking to each other, and adopting this way of life as a preferred alternative to orthodox medical treatment.

I think that it would be worthwhile trying the effect of 'shop-front' facilities in Skid Row areas, providing services that they could make use of if they wished, with the goal of enticing them as voluntary patients into psychiatric treatment.

Patients in mental hospitals

The place of the large mental hospital in psychiatric care should be re-examined. The possibility should be explored that, even after their function as catchment area admission hospitals has ended, they could serve as specialist regional units. Special centres could be based there, for instance units for non-geriatric patients with organic brain disease, alcoholism and drug dependence units, adolescent units, and medium-secure units.

The concept of the 'hospital hostel' should be explored. That is to say a high-dependency hostel, for chronic and disabled patients, situated in the community but close to the DGH psychiatric unit. This is, in essence, a case of transplanting the 'chronic ward' into the catchment area from which the patients originally came. Careful monitoring should assess whether the quality of life is better for patients there than in the 'back ward' of a mental hospital. A controlled trial of the two alternative environments is feasible.

Meanwhile a schedule of desirable standards of care in long-stay wards should be prepared and agreed internationally.

APPENDIX 1

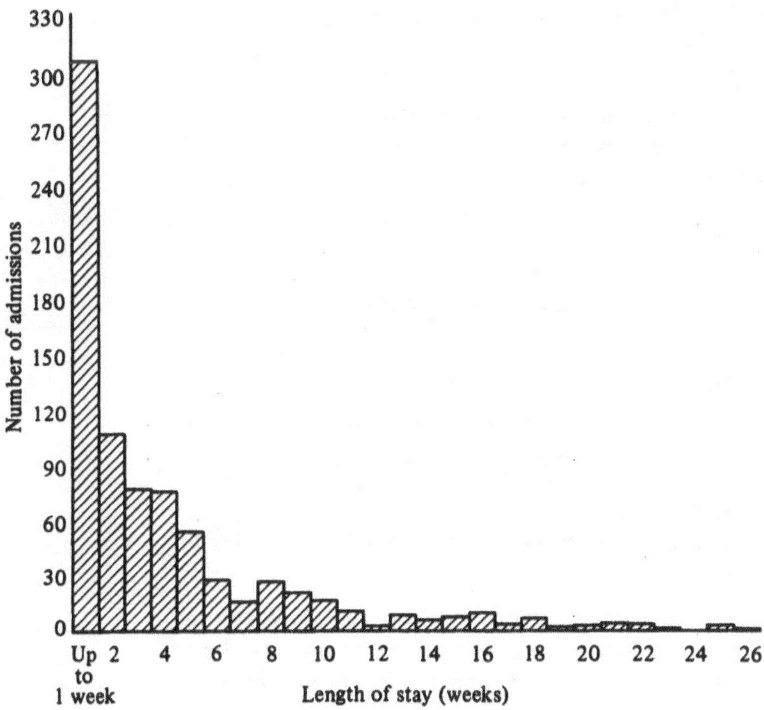

Length of stay of psychiatric patients in a DGH unit.

APPENDIX 2

NAME.......................

DATE.......................

ASSESSMENT OF SOCIAL IMPAIRMENT

Instructions:

Please complete by putting one of the following numbers in the boxes on the right (except questions (9) and (10)):

Yes, definitely	04
Yes, probably	03
Possibly	02
Definitely not	01
Not applicable	−1
Not answered	−2
Not known	−3

Please answer so as to reflect the abilities of the patient on the date that the questionnaire is completed.

Thank you.

Job Capability

(1) Is he capable of carrying out his *usual* job

(2) Is he capable of any employment in the competitive market

(3) Is he capable up to the level (or above) of working in a sheltered workshop

Housing Needs

(4) Is he able to cope with ordinary housing (including flat, digs etc.)

(5) Is he up to the level (or above) required for hostel accommodation (*note:* do not assume any special hostel restrictions, such as that their residents must be in work)

(6) Does he require hospital in-patient care

Other Needs

(7) Does he require *day hospital* care

(8) Does he require at least *day centre* care

(9) The most appropriate residential situation at present for him would be:

Please tick one

01. Psychiatric in-patient status ☐
02. Long-term hostel (supervised) ☐
03. Long-term group home (unsupervised) ☐
04. Short-stay hostel (supervised) ☐
05. Short-stay group home (unsupervised) ☐
06. Some other sheltered situation (please specify . . . .) ☐
07. Living with his family ☐
08. Living alone ☐
09. Other (please specify . . . .) ☐

(10) The most suitable day-time situation at present would be: ☐☐

Please tick one

01. His usual job ☐
02. Another normal job ☐
03. Sheltered workshop ☐
04. Industrial therapy ☐
05. Day centre ☐
06. Day-hospital ☐
07. Psychiatric in-patient ☐
08. Other (please specify . . . .) ☐

COMPLETED BY:

(SIGNATURE). . . . .

NAME (BLOCK LETTERS) . . . .

POSITION. . . . .

References

Anderson, N. (1923). *The Hobo: The Sociology of the Homeless Man*. Chicago: University of Chicago Press.

Crisp, A. H. & Priest, R. G. (1971). Psychoneurotic profiles in middle age: a study of persons aged 40 to 65 registered with a general practitioner. *British Journal of Psychiatry*, **119**, 385–92.

DHSS (1975*a*). *Better Services for the Mentally Ill*. London: Her Majesty's Stationery Office.

DHSS (1975*b*). *Censuses of A. Patients in Mental Illness Hospitals and Units in England & Wales at the end of* 1971. *B. Mental Illness Day Patients in England & Wales at April 1972*. London: Her Majesty's Stationery Office.

Ey, H. (1957). Preface to *Le Clochard: Etude de Psychologie Sociale*, by A. Vexlaird. Paris: Desclee de Brouwer.

Foulds, G. A. (1965). *Personality and Personal Illness*. London: Tavistock Publications.

Foulds, G. A. & Bedford, A. (1975). Hierarchy of classes of personal illness. *Psychological Medicine*, **5**, 181–92.

Foulds, G. A., Bedford, A. & Csapo, K. G. (1975). Class change in the Personal Illness Hierarchy. *British Journal of Psychiatry*, **127**, 316–19.

Foulds, G. A. & Hope, K. (1968). *Manual of the Symptom-Sign Inventory* (*SSI*). London: University of London Press.

Goldberg, D. (1972). *The Detection of Psychiatric Illness by Questionnaire*, Maudsley Monographs, No. 21. London: Oxford University Press.

Gomez, J. & Priest, R. G. (1976). The use of selected questions from the Symptom-Sign Inventory with long-stay psychiatric patients. *British Journal of Psychiatry*, **128**, 595–8.

Guy, W., Gross, M. & Dennis, H. (1967). An alternative to the double-blind procedure. *American Journal of Psychiatry*, **123**, 1505–12.

HMSO (1960). *Homeless Single Persons*. London: Her Majesty's Stationery Office.

Jones, K. A. (1972). *A History of the Mental Health Services*. London: Routledge Kegan Paul.

Kellerman, F. (1983). Surprises in the surgery. *Doctor*, **13**, No. 13, 47.

Priest, R. G. (1969*a*). *Psychiatric Morbidity in Common Lodging Houses: A Study of Prevalence*. Thesis submitted for the degree of M.D., University of London.

Priest, R. G. (1969*b*). The function of thought disorder: A postulate. *British Journal of Psychiatry*, **115**, 959.

Priest, R. G. (1970). Homeless men – U.K. and U.S.A. *Proceedings of the Royal Society of Medicine*, **63**, 441–5.

Priest, R. G. (1971*a*). The Edinburgh Homeless: A psychiatric survey. *American Journal of Psychotherapy*, **25**, 194–213.

Priest, R. G. (1971*b*). The British candidate for termination of pregnancy: a quantified survey of psychiatric referrals. *British Journal of Psychiatry*, **118**, 579–80.

Priest, R. G. (1972*a*). Termination of pregnancy: referrals to a psychiatrist. In *Psychosomatic Medicine in Obstetrics and Gynaecology*, ed. N. Morris, 534–6. Basel: Karger.

Priest, R. G. (1972*b*). The impact of the Abortion Act: a psychiatrist's observations. *British Journal of Psychiatry*, **121**, 293–7.

Priest, R. G. (1975). Review of Wing, Cooper & Sartorius (1974) *The Measurement and Classification of Psychiatric Syndromes*. *Proceedings of the Royal Society of Medicine*, **68**, 466.

Priest, R. G. (1976*a*). The homeless person and the psychiatric services: an Edinburgh survey. *British Journal of Psychiatry*, **128**, 128–36.

Priest, R. G. (1976*b*). A comparative trial of protriptyline and nortriptyline. *Current Medical Research and Opinion*, **3**, 710–15.

Priest, R. G. (1978). The epidemiology of mental illness: Illustrations from the single homeless population. *Psychiatric Journal of the University of Ottawa*, **3**, 27–32.

Priest, R. G. & Crisp, A. H. (1973). Bereavement and psychiatric symptoms: an item analysis. *Psychotherapy and Psychosomatics*, **22**, 166–71.

Priest, R. G. & Netter, P. (1975). Hostility, somatic symptoms and recovery with antidepressants. *International Pharmacopyschiatry*, **10**, 137–41.

Priest, R. G., Raptopoulos, P. & Chan, M. L. (1979). Psychiatric patients: How long do they stay? *Lancet*, **ii**, 40–1.

Priest, R. G,, Shariatmadari, M. E. & Tarighati, Sh. (1973). Affective states in schizophrenia. *British Journal of Social and Clinical Psychology*, **12**, 283–8.

Priest, R. G. & Steinert, J. (1977). *Insanity: A Study of Major Psychiatric Disorders*. Plymouth: Macdonald & Evans.

Priest, R. G., Tarighati, Sh. & Shariatmadari, M. E. (1969). A brief test of organic brain disease: Validation in a mental hospital population. *Acta Psychiatrica Scandinavica*, **45**, 347.

Sims, A. C. P. & Salmons, P. M. (1975). Severity of symptoms in psychiatric out-patients: use of the General Health Questionnaire in hospital and general practice patients. *Psychological Medicine*, **5**, 62–6.

Tooth, G. C. & Brooke, E. M. (1961). Trends in the mental hospital population and their effect on future planning. *Lancet*, **i**, 710–13.

Wing, J. K. & Brown, G. W. (1970). *Institutionalism and Schizophrenia: A Comparative Study of Three Mental Hospitals* 1960–1968. Cambridge University Press.

Wing, J. K., Cooper, J. E. & Sartorius, N. (1974). *The Measurement and Classification of Psychiatric Symptoms*. Cambridge University Press.

Suicides and functional psychoses

N. JUEL-NIELSEN

The changing patterns of suicide in European countries during the last two decades were discussed by a World Health Organization (WHO) Working Group at a meeting in Athens, 29 September–2 October 1981. Some of the conclusions presented in the report (WHO, 1982) provide a useful background for a discussion of the topic of suicides and functional psychoses.

The WHO working group found the following trends in suicide behaviour worthy of further investigations:

1. the rising rates of suicide in most European countries, which have now reached particularly high levels in Hungary and in the northern parts of Yugoslavia;
2. the exceptional decline in rates in England & Wales and in Greece during the last two decades;
3. the relatively low rate in Norway compared with other Scandinavian countries;
4. the marked increase in rates for elderly women in most European countries;
5. the marked increase in rates for young adults in most European countries.

The working group related the changes in reported suicide rates to the social and economic changes in societies that are likely to lead to social isolation of individuals. The following categories were considered high-risk groups for suicide:

1. persons known to be subject to depressive illness,
2. psychiatric hospital in-patients,
3. those who have attempted suicide,
4. alcoholics.

A large number of investigations in various countries have shown that a considerable proportion (at least one third) of those who commit suicide are psychotics: i.e. patients with depressions (with endogenous as well as reactive depressions), schizophrenia or psychoorganic syndromes. Several studies report that 10–15% of manic-depressive patients will end their life by comitting suicide, and a similar suicide risk has been found among schizophrenic patients.

Within recent years a considerable increase in suicide among patients in psychiatric institutions has been reported from Norway, Finland, The Netherlands, UK and other countries. In Norway, the rates were eight times higher in 1970–4 than in 1950–3 (Hessø, 1977; Retterstøl, 1978).

The increasing suicide behaviour in the general population and among psychiatric patients in the Scandinavian countries has given rise to concern, not only among psychiatrists, but also among those responsible for the medical care and social development of the Scandinavian societies.

As a result of this concern the medical research councils in the Nordic countries decided, in 1977, to set up a joint Nordic research project on suicide behaviour. The Nordic Project has primarily been dealing with an analysis of the marked difference between the low suicide rates in Norway (below 10 per 100000) and the high rates (above 20 per 100000) in Finland, Sweden and Denmark.

Preliminary publications (Kolmos, Bach & Hessø, 1983; Retterstøl & Juel-Nielsen, 1983), based on a comparative epidemiological analysis of the ascertainment procedures in Finland, Norway, Sweden and Denmark, confirm the existence of a real difference in the suicide rates within Scandinavia, especially in the younger age groups.

The Nordic project has also included studies of certain high-risk groups (young adults and psychiatric patients, in particular). The reported increase in suicide among psychiatric patients in Norway and in Sweden has caused the National Health Service in these countries to establish a close registration of all suicides in the psychiatric services (O. Rafaelsen, personal communication).

In Denmark, a systematic nationwide registration of suicides among psychiatric patients has not yet been established, but, within the framework of the Nordic Research Project, epidemiological and clinical studies have been performed in an area – the county of Funen – which is assumed to be representative of the Danish society in demographic, economic, social, medical and other respects. The county comprises the island of Funen and some smaller islands and has a population of about 440000, corresponding to 8% of the total population of Denmark.

From a survey (K. Lindekilde & N. Juel-Nielsen, unpublished) of the suicide behaviour in the population in Funen, a few preliminary results are presented in order to answer the following questions:

1. what is the relationship between the increase in suicide in the general population and the increase in suicide among psychiatric patients?; and
2. which diagnostic categories are involved in the latter group?

Fig. 1 presents the absolute number of suicides during the 3-year period 1979–81. The corresponding rates have increased from 23 to 34 per 100000.

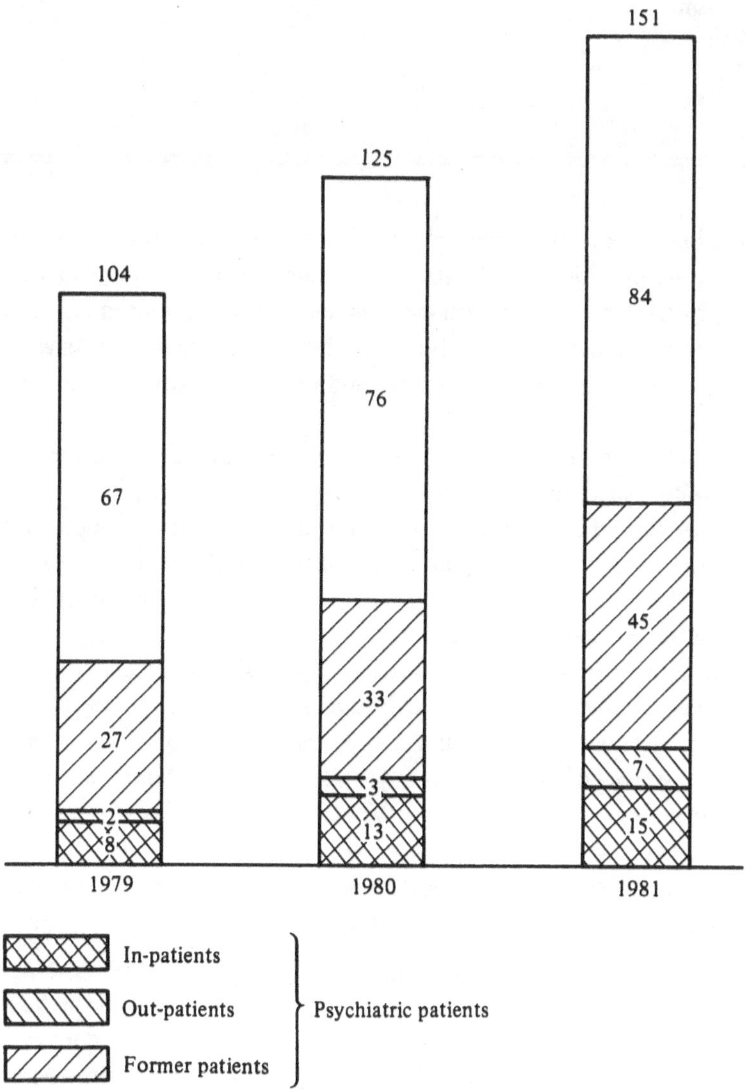

Fig. 1. Absolute number of suicides in the county of Funen (population 440000) 1979–81.

Table 1. *Diagnostic classification of suicides among psychiatric in- and out-patients in the county of Funen 1979–81*

	Number of patients	
Manic-depressive psychosis	15	Psychoses 39 (80%)
Reactive depressive psychosis	12	
Schizophrenia	9	
Organic Syndrome	3	
Alcoholism	3	
Neurosis	3	
Others	3	
Total	48	

Suicide behaviour has increased by 45% in the total population and by 81% among psychiatric patients. The increase is thus considerably higher among psychiatric patients (in-patients as well as out-patients) than the increase among persons who have not been in contact with psychiatric services. These figures confirm the findings in the other Scandinavian studies.

An increase in suicide behaviour in the general population will most likely influence the suicide risk within psychiatric services, but apparently this is not the whole explanation; it should also be mentioned that the decline in suicide rates in England has not been reflected in the psychiatric services, where, on the contrary, hospital statistics show an increase in suicide among resident patients.

Table 1 provides a rough impression of the diagnostic classification of the patients who committed suicide during treatment in the psychiatric services in the county of Funen. As appears, no less than four-fifths of the patients were psychotic and about half of these patients were manic-depressives or schizophrenics. What is the explanation for this development?

The introduction of new methods and principles of treatment in psychiatry has been mentioned by Winokur (1981) who states, that

> if one looks at mental hospital statistics in Finland and Norway, one is immediately struck by the fact that suicides in the hospital populations were at their lowest in the years when a considerable amount of electroconvulsive therapy was used. As electroconvulsive therapy became less used and patients were treated with various drugs, the risk of suicide became greater. However, this

is not the whole story. In those same years, hospitals became increasingly less restricted and more democratic.

Although it seems as if the introduction of the psychopharmacological era (with neuroleptics, antidepressives and drugs with prophylactic properties like lithium) coincides with an increase instead of a decrease in suicides among psychiatric patients, it may be perhaps more relevant that the development of community psychiatry, open-door arrangements, expansion of rehabilitation efforts, extensive use of various psychotherapeutic methods, group therapy etc. has changed the general attitude of the personnel in the psychiatric services towards suicide behaviour. Suicide is often considered to be 'a human right', of which not even the psychotic patient should be deprived; the increasing rate of suicide in the psychiatric services is looked upon as 'a price', which has to be paid for the advantages of a so-called liberal therapeutic policy. Those who favour a viewpoint of this kind seem to ignore the fact that the price is paid by psychiatric patients, primarily psychotic patients suffering from manic-depressive and schizophrenic illness.

The present state of knowledge within the field of prevention of suicide among patients with functional psychoses is incomplete, and further research in multi-centre studies seems to be urgently needed.

References

Hessø, R. (1977). Suicide in Norwegian, Finnish and Swedish psychiatric hospitals. *Archiv für Psychiatrie und Nervenkrankheiten*, **224**, 119–27.

Kolmos, L., Bach, E. & Hessø, R. (1983). The reliability of the Scandinavian suicide rates. In *Depression and Suicide*, ed. J. P. Soubrier & J. Vedrinne, pp. 115–20. Oxford: Pergamon Press.

Retterstøl, N. (1978). Suicide in psychiatric hospitals in Norway. *Psychiatrica Fennica*. Suppl. 89–92.

Retterstøl, N. & Juel-Nielsen, N. (1983). The differences in the Scandinavian rates. In *Depression and Suicide*, ed. J. P. Soubrier & J. Vedrinne, pp. 111–14. Oxford: Pergamon Press.

WHO (1982). *Changing Patterns in Suicide Behaviour*. Report on a WHO Working Group, Athens, 1981. Copenhagen: Regional Office for Europe, WHO.

Winokur, G. (1981). *Depression: The Facts*. Oxford: Oxford University Press.

Interaction with families

J. LEFF

Background

A series of studies has established a strong and replicable relationship between certain emotional attitudes of family members and the outcome of schizophrenia over a period of up to 2 years (Brown *et al.*, 1962; Brown, Birley & Wing, 1972; Vaughn & Leff, 1976*a*; Leff & Vaughn, 1981). To date, this relationship has been established only in the Anglo-Saxon cultures of England and the west coast of America. In these English-speaking samples, the key emotional attitudes of relatives that predict relapse of schizophrenia are criticism and over-involvement. In both the London and California studies, if relatives made six or more critical comments in the course of the interview or scored three or above on the over-involvement scale, the relapse rate for schizophrenia was more than 50% over 9 months. Relatives with scores of this magnitude are categorized as high on expressed emotion (EE). Patients who live with high EE relatives have significantly lower relapse rates if they take regular maintenance anti-psychotic medication or if they are in low face-to-face contact with the relatives, that is, they keep out of their way.

The effectiveness of prophylactic medication is now well established but, until recently it was not known whether the association between high EE and schizophrenic relapse reflected a causal connection; nor was it known whether low face-to-face contact was genuinely protective. Two controlled trials of social intervention in the families of schizophrenic patients living with high EE relatives have been published recently (Falloon *et al.*, 1982; Leff *et al.*, 1982). One trial was carried out in California and involved a behavioural approach to working with the families (Falloon *et al.*, 1982). The other took place in London and evaluated a package of social treatments, including mental health education of the relatives, a relatives' group and family therapy. In both trials, patients were maintained on prophylactic medication. Despite the differences in venue and therapeutic approach, the results of the two trials were remarkably similar. In the California study the relapse rates for the experimental and control groups over 9 months were 6% and 44% respectively, while the comparable figures in the London study were 8% and 50%. Taken together, these results provide evidence for a causal role of relatives' EE in schizophrenic relapse. They also demonstrate the effectiveness of a variety of therapeutic approaches to the family when combined with maintenance drug treatment of the patient. In addition, the study by Leff *et al.* (1982) suggests that lowering face-to-face contact with high EE relatives improves the prognosis for schizophrenic patients.

Suggestions for future research

Schizophrenia

Extension of work on schizophrenia to non-English-speaking cultures

The association between high EE and relapse of schizophrenia has been established only in English-speaking cultures to date. In view of the evidence that the expression of emotion varies from culture to culture (Leff, 1981), there is good reason to repeat the studies in non-English-speaking cultures.

The 2-year follow-up of the International Pilot Study of Schizophrenia (WHO, 1979) demonstrated that the course of schizophrenia was more benign in non-western countries (particularly India and Nigeria) than in the West. One possible explanation is that the level of EE of relatives is lower in more traditional societies, and that this results in a lower relapse rate of schizophrenia. This possibility is currently being explored in a WHO study involving centres in Aarhus, Denmark and in Chandigarh, India. It is already apparent that the North Indian relatives express much less criticism than their Anglo-Saxon counterparts and over-involvement is virtually absent among them. In order for this finding to be taken at its face value it is necessary to ensure that the technique of assessment is transferable across linguistic and cultural barriers. The use of a bilingual rater has demonstrated that this is true of the transfer from English to Hindi (N. N. Wig, D. K. Menon, H. Bedi, A. Ghosh, L. Kuipers, J. Leff, A. Korten, R. Day, N. Sartorius, G. Ernberg, A. Jablensky, unpublished). However the analysis of the follow-up data in this WHO study has not yet been completed, so that it is unknown whether the lower level of EE in Hindi-speaking relatives accounts for the better prognosis of schizophrenic patients.

Further studies of this kind need to be undertaken and the work should be extended to include pre-literate cultures and people who speak languages outside of the Indo-European group.

Evaluation of different therapeutic approaches to altering high EE families.

Both controlled trials of social intervention with high EE families produced similar results, despite the considerable differences in therapeutic approach (Falloon *et al.*, 1982; Leff *et al.*, 1982). This suggests that in these Anglo-Saxon families a variety of types of intervention may be of similar effectiveness in achieving the aims of reduction in relatives' EE and face-to-face contact. Further studies are indicated in which different therapeutic methods of working with families are compared. For example, multiple family groups could be compared with individual families; a behavioural approach could be compared with structural family therapy. In all these studies, cost–benefit analysis should be an essential component; for instance, a relatives' group is much more economical in terms of therapeutic time and therapists' training than family therapy.

Assessment of EE in extra-familial social environments

The work on EE in London has demonstrated that high EE attitudes are not confined to the blood relatives of schizophrenic patients, since high criticism levels have been found in spouses of both schizophrenic and depressed patients (Vaughn & Leff, 1976*a*). Over-involvement has also been found on occasions in both these groups of non-genetic relatives. This evidence suggests that criticism and over-involvement may develop in individuals who are unrelated to the patients either by blood or by marriage. They might be found, for example, among professionals caring for patients in a residential setting, such as a hostel, in non-professionals involved in adult fostering of schizophrenic patients, or in other patients residing in a group home. If this were the case, it would have considerable bearing on the issue of relapse of patients living in sheltered accommodation of a variety of types. This possibility needs to be explored by studies of EE among non-relatives caring for, or living with, schizophrenic patients in sheltered accommodation, and in the follow-up of the patients involved.

Manic-depressive psychosis

Extension of EE studies to mania

It is known that critical attitudes of relatives are not only related to the outcome of schizophrenia, but also to that of depressive neurosis (Vaughn & Leff, 1976*a*) and to successful maintenance of weight loss by obese women (Havstad, 1982). In the latter two conditions, the subjects appeared to be even more sensitive to criticism than schizophrenic patients, since the best discrimination between successful and unsuccessful outcomes was achieved with a level of only two critical comments (cf. six in schizophrenia). It would appear sensible to assess the EE of relatives of manic patients, to determine whether it bears any relationship to outcome of the illness. In the work on schizophrenia, it was found that patients in high contact with high EE relatives had a high relapse rate despite being on regular maintenance drugs. In the same way, a high EE family environment might explain the failure of some manic patients to be controlled by maintenance lithium.

Extension of EE studies to psychotic depression

The argument outlined above also applies to psychotic depression. In the study by Vaughn & Leff (1976*a*) a group of depressed neurotic patients was included and the EE of their relatives assessed. A few patients were identified who lived with non-critical relatives and who had not experienced any life events prior to the onset of their illness. This group of patients could be viewed as suffering from 'endogenous depression' without any obvious environmental precipitants. The criterion for depressive neurosis in this study was the presence of depression without delusions or hallucinations. These patients may represent the tail-end of an endogenous depressive group extending into the clinical sphere of depressive neurosis. From the point of view of the classification of depressive illness, it would be of considerable interest to assess both relatives' EE and the occurrence of life events in patients with psychotic depression, that is depression plus delusions and hallucinations.

Technical issues

Assessment of EE as a clinical tool

For some time we have been aware of the necessity of bringing the assessment of relatives' EE within the reach of the clinical team. Our first step was to streamline the original lengthy interview of Brown & Rutter (1966) to 1 hour's duration without losing any of the discrimination ability of the technique (Vaughn & Leff, 1976*b*). However, assessment of EE requires careful listening to the tape-recorded interview, which usually occupies a further 1.5 hours. This amount of time places a considerable burden on the busy clinical team, particularly when it is appreciated that the training for EE assessment takes at least 3 weeks, full-time.

The two trials of social intervention referred to earlier indicate that every clinical team dealing with schizophrenic patients needs to be able to identify high EE families. To this end, it is essential to develop a brief method of assessing EE, which might not be as sensitive as the research technique, but would become a practical clinical tool.

Relationship between EE and other assessment techniques

EE is by no means the only measure of family functioning which has been shown to be linked with the outcome of schizophrenia. Affective style (Doane *et al.*, 1981) and the Revealed Differences Technique (Strodtbeck, 1951; Angermeyer, 1982) are two examples of alternative approaches. It would be of great interest to determine whether these techniques all tap the same aspect of family functioning, or whether there is little, if any, overlap between them. To determine this, it would be necessary to employ two or more methods of assessment of the same families.

References

Angermeyer, M. C. (1982). The association between family atmosphere and hospital career of schizophrenic patients. *British Journal of Psychiatry*, **141**, 1–11.

Brown, G. W., Birley, J. L. T. & Wing, J. K. (1972). Influence of family life on the course of schizophrenic disorders: a replication. *British Journal of Psychiatry*, **121**, 241–58.

Brown, G. W., Monck, E. M., Carstairs, G. M. & Wing, J. K. (1962). Influence of family life on the course of schizophrenic illness. *British Journal of Preventive and Social Medicine*, **16**, 55–68.

Brown, G. W. & Rutter, M. (1966). The measurement of activities and relationships: a methodological study. *Human Relations*, **19**, 241–63.

Doane, J. A., West, K. L., Goldstein, M. J., Rodnick, E. A. & Jones, J. E. (1981). Parental affective style and communication deviance as predictors of subsequent schizophrenia spectrum disorders in vulnerable adolescents. *Archives of General Psychiatry*, **38**, 679–85.

Falloon, I. R. H., Boyd, J. L., McGill, C. W., Razani, J., Moss, H. B. & Gilderman, A. M. (1982). Family management in the prevention of exacerbations of schizophrenia: a controlled study. *New England Journal of Medicine*, **306**, 1437–40.

Havstad, L. F. (1982). Weight loss and weight loss maintenance as aspects of family emotional processes. Ph.D. thesis, University of Southern California.

Leff, J. P. (1981). *Psychiatry Around the Globe: A Transcultural View*. New York: Dekker.

Leff, J., Kuipers, L., Berkowitz, R., Eberlein-Vries, R. & Sturgeon, D. (1982). A controlled trial of social intervention in the families of schizophrenic patients. *British Journal of Psychiatry*, **141**, 121–34.

Leff, J. & Vaughn, C. (1981). The role of maintenance therapy and relatives' expressed emotion in relapse of schizophrenia: a two-year follow-up. *British Journal of Psychiatry*, **139**, 102–4.

Strodtbeck, F. L. (1951). Husband–wife interaction over revealed differences. *American Sociological Review*, **16**, 468–73.

Vaughn, C. & Leff, J. (1976*a*). The influence of family and social factors on the course of psychiatric illness: a comparison of schizophrenic and depressed neurotic patients. *British Journal of Psychiatry*, **129**, 125–37.

Vaughn, C. & Leff, J. (1976*b*). The measurement of expressed emotion in families of psychiatric patients. *British Journal of Social and Clinical Psychology*, **15**, 157–65.

World Health Organization (1979). *Schizophrenia: an International Follow-up Study*. Chichester: John Wiley.

Cost-effectiveness analysis

D. GOLDBERG

In a traditional cost-effectiveness analysis there is a single objective which is usually measured by a common physical unit (i.e. number of breast cancers detected, number of chronic schizophrenics who return to full employment), and we want to achieve either a fixed level of objective at minimum cost, or as much objective as we can for a fixed cost. There is, therefore, some sort of outcome which is explicitly stated for each service or method of treatment, and the analysis will compare the cost of achieving the goal by various means. It is not easy to find examples of such analyses in psychiatry, since it is unusual to think of the effectiveness of treatment in such crude terms. Patients who have received a particular treatment cannot be usefully divided into 'still ill' and 'cured'; and indeed we may wish to examine the effects of a particular treatment on many different aspects of psychosocial adjustment. It is also sometimes necessary to evaluate services which do not reduce disability at all: for example, services for mentally handicapped children, or for severely demented old people. Fortunately, it is possible to modify cost-effectiveness analysis in such a way that useful conclusions about psychiatric services can still be drawn.

The basic strategy of such modified studies is to compare two alternative forms of treatment service as comprehensively as possible in terms of the quality of care provided and the effects which they have on their patients. No attempt should be made to express the value of these effects in monetary terms. An overall comparison is made of all the ways in which these two services compare with one another, and this is examined to see whether one service is clearly superior to the other, or whether no clear superiority emerges. The economic analysis is carried out separately, and addresses itself to what each service costs. A service which is more expensive than another should be able to justify the increased cost in terms of the higher quality of the services provided. A cost-effectiveness analysis provides us with a rough framework for effecting a comparison between expenditure on health care and the quality of the resulting service.

The essence of any evaluation is a comparison between two alternative forms of treatment service, or between a new form of service and an established form.

Stated in this general form, it is evident that cost-effectiveness analysis covers a wide range of evaluative studies ranging from very simple comparisons on the one hand to highly complex controlled studies with prospective random assignment of patients on the other. For example, we might compare the quality of care available in two different kinds of childrens' home in terms of quite simple indicators such as the quality of the buildings, the range of activities available for the children, the childrens' overall level of physical and psychological health, and the satisfaction of the children and their relatives with the care received. These qualitative differences between the homes would be offset against the cost of providing each service in terms of capital and revenue expenditure. Such a study could be carried out on a low budget by a trained research worker, and would not be especially time consuming. Although modest, such a study might enable firm conclusions to be drawn concerning a particular pattern of service.

At the other extreme are complex designs used to evaluate programmes for particular diseases which may have far-reaching economic consequences. If the economic analysis is extended to cover benefits as well as costs then these more complex comparisons are best described as 'modified cost–benefit analysis', since a comprehensive comparison of two services in non-monetary terms is then considered together with a conventional cost–benefit analysis (Williams, 1974; Glass & Goldberg, 1977). An example of such a study would be the Manchester Schizophrenia Study (Goldberg & Jones, 1980; Jones, Goldberg & Hughes, 1980). This study compared the services offered by an area mental hospital and the psychiatric unit of a district general hospital by following two groups of first admission schizophrenics admitted to each service. The patients were compared in terms of the services used over the course of 1 year, and the investigators measured the clinical and social adjustment of the patients, and the effects that the patients' illnesses had on their families. The economic analysis was not confined merely to costs of the patients' psychiatric care, but included all cash flows caused by the patients' illnesses, from the viewpont first of the rest of the community, and second from that of the patients' families. It was possible to bring all these financial effects together in the form of a single 'net effect' which represents the overall financial comparison between the services.

Levels of complexity of the economic analysis

The simplest type of evaluation is confined to the direct psychiatric health costs of the treatment services. May's classic cost-effectiveness study, which compared different treatments for acute schizophrenia, merely considered the costs of various components of hospital care (May, 1971); but Mancini and Burchell's comparison between mental hospital and the Maudsley hostel ward in the treatment of the new long-stay patient considered the costs per patient day in the two services, and also compares the capital costs. It emerged in the latter study that the hostel ward was cheaper in terms of capital costs, but rather more expensive in terms of revenue costs: mainly because of the costs of paramedical supporting services and general services at this particular hostel. (The study is briefly referred to in Wing & Wykes, 1982; full details from the Economic Adviser's Office, DHSS, London.)

Simple cost comparisons such as these are justifiable where the evaluation is being undertaken entirely from the viewpoint of the health providers, or where the patients receiving the service are not likely *either* to engage in open employment *or* to have adverse economic effects on other members of their families. If these conditions are not met, it is unwise to undertake such a simple economic analysis, since it is known that the indirect costs of psychiatric illness greatly exceed the direct costs.

An intermediate level of economic analysis is concerned with *general costs*, not merely of the psychiatric services, but also including general health costs, family doctor costs, local authority welfare services costs, social security payments and rent rebates, and travel costs. An example would be Mangen *et al.*'s comparison between hospital out-patient services and community psychiatric nurses in the treatment of depression: here the total costs were 8–10 times higher than the psychiatric costs, and there was no overall difference between the services in economic terms. This study was superior in that it used prospective random assignment of patients to the two treatment services, but it was limited in that it did not measure economic benefits in the form of the patient's earnings (Mangen *et al.*, 1983).

The most ambitious designs attempt to measure all the cash flows caused by illness from the standpoint of the patient and his family on the one hand, and the rest of the community on the other. Thus it also records loss of earnings by family members who have had to stop work to look after the patient, extra earnings by family members obliged to work to help provide for the patient, as well as the earnings of the patients themselves. Such detailed studies are time consuming and demanding, and can only be meaningful if the two groups of patients are exactly comparable in type of mental illness, chronicity of illness, and socioeconomic status. (It is obvious that if service 'A' treats minor disorders in those with high income, it will be economically superior to service 'B' that treats unemployed people with chronic psychoses and organic states; that will be true *however* the two services are organized.)

If we now apply these arguments to the evaluation of treatment services for those with long-term functional psychoses, we see that in the case of a comparison between two essentially institutional forms of treatment the simplest form of economic analysis will be adequate, but if one service is community based it will be necessary to use at least an intermediate form of analysis. Finally, if either service is successful in returning patients to open employment it will be necessary to include data relating to earnings, since these are likely to make a substantial contribution to an overall economic evaluation.

Levels of complexity of the non-monetary evaluation

The unthinking investigator measures everything in sight: symptoms of illness, disabilities and defects consequent upon illness, social adjustment of the patient – all these in both the patient and his living group – as well as characteristics of the treatment services themselves. Unless the investigator has no idea about the likely non-monetary benefits of a particular service, it is undoubtedly better to concentrate the evaluation on those aspects of outcome that are likely to be affected. In the Manchester Schizophrenia Study for example, there were fewer defect states in the community oriented service, and the patients' social adjustment was also superior. Scales measuring disabilities, defects and social adjustment are particularly relevant in the assessment of services for ambulant psychotic patients discharged in the community. In Wing & Wykes' hostel ward comparison however, where the patients in the comparison were all institutionalized, the evaluation included a patient's attitude scale and a time budget as well as a social adjustment scale, since it was anticipated that the new service might produce advantages in these areas. (Most investigators include symptom scales as outcome measures in such studies but it is unusual to find any differences between groups providing they were carefully matched *ab initio*; however there may well be differences in the mean dosage of neuroleptics required to achieve minimal symptom levels.)

Although it is usual to evaluate treatment services by measuring the effects that they have on two groups of comparable patients, it is worth remembering that there are some useful indicators of the quality of service that can be obtained very much more simply by clinically inexperienced research workers.

Indicators of quality

Below are listed those indicators of quality which can be obtained easily in a comparison between two services:

1. Waiting time to be seen in the clinic,
2. quality of buildings and furnishings,
3. efficiency and courtesy of receptionists and clinic nurses,
4. adequacy of training of paramedical staff,
5. availability and use of a wide range of treatments (medical, psychological and social),
6. extent of undesirable practices (e.g. physical restraint, seclusion rooms, excessive electroconvulsive therapy, excessive use of compulsory powers, over-sedation),
7. extent of desirable practices (e.g. accessibility and friendliness of staff, frequency with which patient is seen by qualified staff), and
8. full range of rehabilitation facilities freely available.

There are some *additional indicators that could only be assessed by clinically experienced independent research workers:*

9. thoroughness of assessment interview,
10. quality of doctor's interview skills,
11. sophistication of formulations, adequacy of notes, and
12. appropriateness of treatment offered.

It is not clear that the latter group of indicators would add very much to the information more easily obtained by the first eight, and they would undoubtedly be more difficult to obtain. It is interesting to notice that client-satisfaction is likely to be determined by a group of indicators different from those which determine clinical and economic effectiveness: indeed, 'waiting time' is probably the only indicator that is related to all three. Client satisfaction is likely to be determined by indicators 1, 2, 3 and 7, and perhaps by 6. Economic effectiveness is likely to be largely determined by 1, 5 and 12, with other factors being only related indirectly. Finally, clinical effectiveness is not likely to be much affected by indicators 2 and 3, but is otherwise determined by the widest range of indicators.

It should not be forgotten that a good evaluation should include a systematic description of the two services that are being compared, and that some of the indicators mentioned are themselves necessarily indicative of the quality of the services being compared.

Some methodological problems

It follows from what has been said that when we compare two services we are necessarily comparing two treatment packages. These are typically forms of service that are appropriate in the country concerned, but which offer a number of points of contrast with one another. Unfortunately if one service is clearly superior to the other, we still do not know which component or components were responsible for the difference between them. We can sometimes do a within-group analysis to see whether those patients who did particularly well with the superior service tended to use a particular component that was not available in the other service; but the results of such analyses will be suggestive rather than conclusive. The problem can only be solved by carrying out more comparisons in which we choose the services in such a way that the components are varied one at a time. This reminds us of the importance of *replication* in evaluation research: we need to know if our findings hold up across diagnoses, across social and cultural settings, and for treatment packages which have many different combinations of characteristics. If the model for evaluation is too elaborate and time consuming, we shall never obtain the number of evaluative studies that are necessary to obtain reliable results.

It must be remembered that a comparison between two services can only tell us which service is preferable: it cannot say whether there is not some other way of running a service that would be far more effective than either, or indeed whether it is worth having any service at all. Another problem is likely to arise if investigators choose large numbers of non-monetary measures of the quality of service: the higher the number, the more likely it is that some of them will point in one direction, and some in another. The results can only be interpreted if one service is clearly superior to the other. If investigators clearly state the aim of a particular service, and devise a small number of outcome measures that are addressed to that aim, interpretation of results is likely to be straightforward.

A number of problems commonly arise with the economic analysis. If psychiatric patients are treated in a general hospital, it is difficult to obtain even specialty costings (i.e. the cost of treating a *psychiatric* patient) without making many arbitrary assumptions concerning the extent to which the psychiatry department uses various services within the hospital, and it is extremely difficult to calculate disease costings (i.e. the cost of treating, for example, a schizophrenic patient on a ward containing patients with many other illnesses). Such costings require a special observational study. Next, the appropriate cost to use is the 'long run marginal cost', but this is often impossible to calculate, so that average costs have to be used instead. Finally, we are tempted to carry out our evaluations over short time periods, yet we know that treatments for chronic psychotic patients may exert profound economic consequences spread over long periods of time. Thus a treatment which is expensive and appears economically disadvantageous in the short term may be the best treatment in the long term. There are methods of economic analysis which make allowance for such effects ('discounting'): our problem is that we are tempted to draw conclusions from studies that have only been funded to run for 2 or 3 years.

Areas in which further research is needed

We have argued that some problems in evaluation can be carried out with simple research designs, so that elaborate modified cost–benefit models are reserved for studies where some of the patients will be returning to employment, and where it is thought necessary to ascribe all the economic consequences of illness. It is axiomatic that one should choose the simplest model that is adequate for a particular comparison, and one should consider separately the economic and the non-monetary effects when making this choice. It should not be thought that once two types of service have been compared the problem is solved: evaluations need to be replicated in different places with services that will inevitably have somewhat different combinations of characteristics.

New patterns of services need to be compared with traditional patterns. The fewer the points of contrast between the two services, the easier it will be to interpret the results. The task of a researcher who has skills in evaluation is not to invent some new service, but to offer to evaluate an existing service that differs in some important respect from the traditional service. (Good researchers and gifted innovators are seldom the same people.)

Each contributor to this volume will have his own list of evaluations that should be made in his or her country. Here is mine:

A. For 'new long stay' patients comparisons should be made between:

1. care in hospital wards and care in 'hostel wards';
2. regimens in hostel wards where the day is spent in workshops, and regimens where the day is spent in domestic tasks such as shopping, cooking, cleaning, decorating and gardening;
3. regimens which make extensive use of rehabilitation workshops and those which do not, with special attention to the stage of the illness in which the rehabilitative effort is made;
4. hostel wards which make extensive use of behavioural treatment methods and those which do not.

B. For ambulant chronic psychotic patients comparisons should be made between:

1. traditional regimens which allow admissions whenever clinical relapse occurs, and those which use community psychiatric nurses and community workers to discourage readmissions;
2. traditional regimens which aim rehabilitation at either open employment or sheltered workshop employment, and those which pioneer leisure activities which do not mimic the activities of employed people, but which are nonetheless goal-orientated and structured;
3. various types of living accommodation for chronic psychotic patients estranged from their families (it would be particularly valuable to have a comparison between forms of residential care where supervision is provided by professional care-givers, and forms of care where patients themselves are responsible for befriending one another, perhaps with assistance from a community psychiatric nurse);
4. regimens which make extensive use of attendance at day-hospital facilities and those where the patients stay at home and are visited by CPNs.

References

Glass, N. J. & Goldberg, D. (1977). Cost-benefit analysis and the evaluation of psychiatric services. *Psychological Medicine*, **7**, 701–7.

Goldberg, D. & Jones, R. (1980). The costs and benefits of psychiatric care. In *The Social Consequences of Psychiatric Illness*, ed. L. N. Robins, P. J. Clayton & J. K. Wing. New York: Brunner/Mazel, Inc.

Jones, R., Goldberg, D. & Hughes, B. (1980). A comparison of two different services treating schizophrenia: a cost–benefit approach. *Psychological Medicine*, **10**, 493–505.

Mangen, S. P., Paykel, E. S., Griffith, J. H., Burchell, A. & Mancini, P. (1983). Cost-effectiveness of community psychiatric nurse or out-patient psychiatric care of neurotic patients. *Psychological Medicine*, **13**, 407–17.

May, P. R. A. (1971). Cost-efficiency of treatments for the schizophrenic patient. *American Journal of Psychiatry*, **127**(10), 1382–5.

Williams, A. (1974). The cost benefit approach. *British Medical Bulletin*, **30**(3), 252–6.

Wing, J. & Wykes, J. (1982). Long-term community care: experience in a London Borough. *Psychological Medicine*, Monograph Suppl. **2**, 59–97.

Consumption of services – European aspects

J. H. HENDERSON

Introduction

The Mental Health Programme of the World Health Organization (WHO) has, for 10 years, been promoting a consistent policy for the development of mental health services. This policy is one based upon the provision of comprehensive community-based mental health care. In this, the principal features are unequivocal. The size of large mental hospitals should be reduced; alternative in-patient treatment facilities should be provided (preferably within general hospitals alongside other medical specialities); residential care should be as near to the population it serves as possible; out-patient and day care facilities should be available wherever patients needs can be met without admission to hospital; non-medical extramural care by nurses, social workers and the like should be developed; and mental health personnel should work as much as possible in multi-disciplinary teams, serving defined populations.

Many of these essential policy elements are not measurable in strict statistical terms, but some can be translated into indicators or measures of identifiable trends. Some possible indicators are presented in this chapter; these are derived partly from data presently available at a macro-level, from a selection of countries in Europe. From data available at a micro-level, some detail of the use of services by long-term psychotic patients is shown.

Indicators of trends

A reduction in the number of mental hospitals with more than 1000 beds

Although in inter-country comparison, there is some difficulty in defining what a mental hospital is, there is no difficulty thereafter in identifying those institutions which contain more than 1000 beds. It is an

Table 1. *Number of mental hospitals with more than 1000 beds by country*

	1972	1982
Italy	55	20
United Kingdom	65	31
Spain	14	nil
Sweden	10	4
Czechoslovakia	6	nil
Total for 19 countries	232	97

assumption however that where the size of these hospitals has decreased, some alternative modes of care have been developed.

In the 19 countries for which we have comparable data on mental hospitals, there was a total of 232 mental hospitals of over 1000 beds in 1972 which had diminished to only 97 hospitals by 1982. Five hospitals with over 2000 beds were reported in 1972, but none existed 10 years later. Italy (with a reduction from 55 to 20 large hospitals) and the United Kingdom (with a reduction from 65 to 31) provide striking examples. In the other 17 countries there was a total of 112 large mental hospitals in 1972 and only 46 in 1982. As a measure of progress then we can record that throughout Europe, during the 10 years, there was a reduction of between one half and two thirds in the number of large mental hospitals.

Increase in general hospital units

The corollary in service development of a reduction in the number of beds in psychiatric hospitals is an increase in the number of beds in general hospitals or in other convenient community settings. The development of psychiatric units in general hospitals has the main virtue of bringing psychiatry and the treatment of psychiatric illness into the same orbit as other medical specialties. It reduces the risks and ill effects of labelling and stigma, facilitates better contact and more cooperation between doctors of different specialties and should improve treatment facilities in the many cases where physical and psychological components both occur in the same patient.

The data available for general hospitals units are far from complete for many countries. Only 15 countries can be compared in 1982 with data from 1972. For these 15 countries the total number of general hospital units in 1972 was 373; this had become 608 by 1982 (an increase of 63%). The total number of beds in general hospital units in these countries had gone up

Table 2. *Numbers of psychiatric beds in general hospitals in 15 countries*

	1972	1982
Total beds	22822	29680
Number of units	374	608
Mean size	61.2	48.8

Table 3. *Highest and lowest country ratios of psychiatric beds per 100000 population*

	1972	1982
Highest	580.2	421.7
Lowest	50	84

from 22822 to 29680 (an increase of 30%) and the mean size of these units had fallen from 61.2 beds to 48.8 beds. The percentage of all psychiatric beds which were in general hospital units had increased from 8.4% to 9.3% but this still remains a very small percentage of the whole. Although this is a fairly crude indicator, it does suggest that there has been some significant advance in the development of general-hospital based units for psychiatry in Europe, but in-patient care is still strongly dominated by the traditional mental hospital.

Psychiatric beds per 1000 population

This is a complex indicator since it is not at all obvious that more beds per 1000 population is representative of a better psychiatric service. Indeed, the evidence available would suggest that high bed ratios are likely to be associated with many large mental hospitals and a lack of alternatives to in-patient care.

These data are available for most of the countries of Europe and we can compare 28 countries. Both in 1972 and 1982, the range is very considerable, but it has contracted a little. In the earlier survey it varied from 0.2 beds per 1000 to 5.8 beds per 1000. In 1982, the two countries which a decade earlier provided less than 0.5 beds per 1000 maintain this level, while there is a contraction at the top of the range to 4.2 beds per 1000. While in 1972 there were 5 countries with more than 3 beds per 1000 only 3 countries reported more than 3 beds per 1000 in 1982.

Increases in alternatives to in-patient care

Traditionally, in-patient care has dominated the psychiatric services in most countries. Developments in psychiatric care may therefore be measured, albeit somewhat crudely, by increases in out-patient care. Developments in day care too may be used for the same measure. Whereas most countries reported developments in out-patient units of varying kinds, only 13 countries reported developments in day facilities. The overall data in this section, however, were very inadequate and reflected rather the need for a major international commitment to agreements for studies on definition of the many alternatives to in-patient care now being developed and used throughout Europe.

Number of psychiatrists per 100000 population

The data show very high ratios of psychiatrists in many countries in Europe in 1972, which became even greater by 1982. Of 31 countries providing data in 1972, 15 had over 4 psychiatrists per 100000 (though none exceeded 8 per 100000). By 1982, of 23 countries providing suitable data, 16 had over 4 psychiatrists per 100000 and, of these, 6 had over 8 per 100000. The mean for each of these groups was 4.03 per 100000 in 1972 and 6.9 in 1982. The range in 1972 was from 0.1 per 100000 to 7.6, but by 1982 the range was from 0.23 to over 15. If we examine the 21 countries which can be compared between 1972 and 1982, the mean changed from 4.24 per 100000 to 7.04 per 100000.

Experiences from pilot study areas in Europe

A pilot study of mental health services in 21 pilot areas in 16 countries in Europe examined cohorts of 200 consecutive psychiatric patients who had had no contact with the mental health services during the 6 months prior to entry into the cohort. These patients were aged 15 years and over and were collected in the period 1979 to 1980 and followed for a period of 2 years.

From a selection of nine different pilot areas the percentage of psychotic patients within the nine cohorts varied widely from 15% to 62%. The measure of in-patient days for patients diagnosed as psychotic ranged from 5.8 to 157, an incredible variation in the pattern of use of services.

In a further examination and analysis the number of out-patient contacts made by these psychotic patients during a 2-year period was calculated. Again, a wide range of experience was reported from a very low rate of contact (on average 2.6 episodes in the 2 years) to an exceptionally high rate of contact (35.4 episodes during the 2-year period). A further analysis of the numbers of days in day-hospital care is on the

Table 4. *Cohort study results from 9 Pilot Areas*

Pilot Area	1	2	3	4	5	6	7	8	9
Total number in cohort with diagnosis of psychosis	82	191	122	101	91	42	43	32	29
Portion of total cohort (%)	29	37	62	29	46	21	24	16	15
Mean number of in-patient days during 2 years	50.2	123.3	157.0	104.3	12.0	75.0	65.5	39.0	5.8
Mean number of out-patient contacts during 2 years	5.2	8.3	11.0	8.0	35.4	5.7	2.6	8.0	10.7
Mean number of day hospital contacts during 2 years	6.1	24.2	12.9	0.9	20.8	—	3.3	—	7.7

whole seen to be quite low, in the range of 0.2 episodes to 12.9, with one exception in the high range of 24.2.

In this study, the diagnostic grouping of psychotic patients included organic psychoses, schizophrenia, affective psychoses and others. It is by reason of the small numbers of some of these categories that a more detailed breakdown and analysis of more discrete diagnostic groups has not been carried out. Also it is true that, in some areas, patients may have received care from and in agencies or services not covered by the pilot area study.

Nevertheless, this presentation of the experiences of the broad category of psychotic patients does give some measure of the widely varying patterns and use of services by the category of patients most likely to contain the majority of cases of long-term functional psychoses in different centres in different countries in Europe.

Conclusions

The implications for needed research in the area of long-term treatment of functional psychosis, from the results of experiences with two international studies, are manifold.

Of critical importance at the national, or macro-level, is the need to improve mental health information systems in most countries in Europe. A standardized data set for annual completion and submission to the World Health Organization would be a desirable ideal.

In this context an internationally agreed glossary and definition of terms such as in-patient, day-patient, out-patient, mental hospital, general hospital, day hospital, etc. is a necessary prerequisite.

From such simple beginnings, under international agreements a useful recording and reporting system could then be built, covering trends, evaluating and monitoring patterns of care and setting indicators and criteria for measuring change, so essential in dealing with rapidly changing care systems such as those for long-term functional psychosis.

Acknowledgements

The kind assistance of many collaborators in the Member States of the World Health Organization (WHO) European Region is gratefully acknowledged in making available useful data. The work of Dr Hugh Freeman and Dr Tom Fryers in the assessment of the WHO Long-term mental health programme for 1972 to 1982 in the Region provided a wealth of detail for this paper. The data analysis for the WHO study of Mental Health Services in Pilot Study Areas in Europe was done by Professor R. Giel and Dr P. Hermann and their associates and to them also go grateful acknowledgements.

INDEX

Aarhus County psychiatric case register, 199
Aberdeen psychiatric case register, 199
acute schizophrenic episode, classification of, 11
adolescents, psychotic
  community houses, 142
  crisis centres, 142
  treatment of, 141–2
adrenaline
  brain, effect of MAOIs on, 118–19
  CSF values in depression, 118
affective disorders, long-stay population with, 185 (Fig. 1)
affective psychoses (*see also* depression *and* manic-depressive psychosis)
  admissions, in Norway, 17 (Table 2)
  age-related incidence rates, 177–8
  classification of, 11–12
  optimum duration of long-term treatment, 52–3
  psychotherapy for, 53
affective style, 245
affective symptoms in mental illness, 223–4
aggression, anger and psychotic relapse, 94
aging (*see also* elderly)
  of chronic psychotics, 148–9
  effect on brain of, 149
  of schizophrenics, 148–9; and rehabilitation potential, 159
Albenga, case register studies in, 40–3
alcohol-related disorders, long-stay patients, 185 (Fig. 1)
alcoholics
  admissions of, in Norway, 16, 17 (Table 2)
  care facilities for, 29
alcoholism in homeless men, 225
ambulant chronic psychotics, research needed on, 254
ambulatory treatment for psychotic children, 140, 141
amitriptyline, efficacy of, 116
anger, aggression and psychotic relapse, 94
antidepressants (*see also* monoamine oxidase inhibitors)
  cyclic, 120
  inducing psychoses in old age, 148
  long-term treatment with, 52, 108
antiepileptic drugs for manic-depressive psychosis, 108, 109
antipsychotic drugs (*see also* neuroleptic drugs)
  long-term treatment with, 53–4
  for manic-depressive psychosis, 108
anxiety
  role in infanto-juvenile psychosis, 139
  symptoms of, in mental illness, 223–4

Bannister's Repertory Grid Test, 67–8
Beck's cognitive therapy, 65
beds, psychiatric, *see* psychiatric beds
behavioural therapies, 60, 64–7
  cognitive therapy, *see* cognitive therapy
  time out from positive reinforcement (TO), 64
  token economies, 67
benzamides, 103
Bouffées délirantes, 11
brain
  aging of, 145–6, 149
  damage in schizophrenia, 72
  neurotransmitters, and MAOIs, 118–19
brain syndromes, long-stay patients, 185 (Fig. 1)

Camberwell psychiatric case register, 198
carbamazepine for manic-depressive psychosis, 109
Cardiff psychiatric case register, 199

case registers, 197–205
comparability of, 199, 201
cost-effectiveness of psychiatric services and, 205
currently operating in Europe, 198–200
Data Protection Laws and, 200–1
elements of, 197–8
family studies of HLAs, 205
limitations of, 180, 202
Oxford record linkage project, 198
studies in Italy, 40–5
usefulness of, 201–2, 205
WHO European pilot study areas, 205
census investigations
in Norway, 17–18 (Table 3)
usefulness of, 23
children
competence training, 71–2
psychotherapy as prophylaxis in, 71–2
psychotic, 139–41; treatment of, 140–1
chlorpromazine, 103
chronic illness
and changes in health care policy, 178–81
definition of, 210
increasing prevalence of, 178
rising incidence of, 177–8
chronic psychotics (*see also* long-term patients *and* schizophrenia, chronic)
affective symptoms in, 224
aging of, 148–9
ambulant, research needs, 254
behavioural therapies for, 64–7
continuity of care, problems of, 221
homelessness among, 218, 225–6
'hospital hostels' for, 227
neglect of, 217–31
provision of care for, 30–6, 179, 220–1
psychometric testing, 222–4
quality of life of, *see* quality of life
chronicity, 'code' of, 160
classification of functional psychoses, 9–13
clomipramine for depression in general practice, 12
clorgyline, selectivity of, 117
clozapine, 103
cognitive disorders and social relationships, 172–3, 209
cognitive therapy, 64–7
Beck's, 65
rational-emotive therapy, 64
self-instructional training, 64–5, 66
social skills training, 66–7, 127
token economies, 67
committal, *see* compulsory admissions
communications technology and treatment adherence in chronic psychotics, 69
community care (*see also* out-patient care *and* rehabilitation), 54–5
aims of, 192
burden on relatives of, 195
cost-effectiveness analysis of, 250
costs of, 195
development of services, in Italy, 47, 48, 49
evaluation of, 180–1; for chronic schizophrenia, 183–95
patterns of utilization by schizophrenics, 190–4 (Table 3, Figs. 5–7)
planning, 221
policy on, 180
in United Kingdom, 220
community centres, in Italy, 49
community houses for psychotic adolescents, 142
Community Mental Health Centers (USA), 33
community psychiatric nurses, costs of, compared with out-patient services, 249
competence training for children, 71–2
compliance
lithium prophylaxis, 110–11
with psychotherapy research protocol, 70
compulsory admissions
in Italy, 48
length of stay, 34
in Norway, 17
rights of patients and, 60
computerized axial tomography in schizophrenia, 72
Cooper's taxonomic hierarchy for the classification of disability, 212–13, 214–15
cost–benefit analysis, modified, 248
cost–effectiveness analysis, 247–54
case registers, use of, 205
economic analysis, levels of complexity of, 249–50
further research needs, 253–4
indicators of quality, 251
methodological problems, 252–3
non-monetary evaluation, levels of complexity of, 250–1
crisis centres for psychotic adolescents, 142
cyclic antidepressants, 120

Danish in-patient case register, 199
Data Protection Laws and psychiatric case registers, 200–1
day care facilities in Europe, 258
day centres in United Kingdom, 220

day hospitals
  for psychotic children, 140, 141
  utilization of: in Europe, 258–60 (Table 4); in West Germany, 190 (Table 3)
dehospitalization, 4
deinstitutionalization, 4, 27–8
  and provision of community care services, 29, 54
  uncontrolled, problems of, 32
delusional states (*see also* paranoid states)
  in old age, classification of, 147
  treatment of, 54
delusions, systematized, cognitive therapy for, 65–6
Delusions-Symptoms-States Inventory (DSSI), 222
dementia, life expectancy in, 178
demographic changes and prevalence of chronic illness, 177–8
Denmark
  psychiatric case registers, 199
  suicide behaviour in Funen county, 236–8 (Fig. 1, Table 1)
depot-preparations, 103
deprenaline (Deprenyl), selectivity of, 117
depression
  age-related incidence rates, 178
  atypical, and its response to antidepressants, 116–17
  brain neurotransmitters in, 118–19
  costs of treatment services for, 249
  endogeneous: effect of aging on, 148; in general practice, 12; and involutional depression, 147
  expressed emotion of relatives, 244
  involutional, 147
  neurotic: classification of, 12; critical attitudes of relatives in, 243, 244
  phenelzine for, 117
  senile, 147
  symptoms in mental illness, 223–4
depressive states, classification of, 12
diagnosis
  and classification of functional psychoses, 9–13
  problems of, 10–11
  psychometric testing, 223
Diagnosis and Treatment Services (DTS) in Italy, 47, 48, 49
diagnostic systems, development of, 103
diazepam for neurotic patients, 116
digitalis inducing psychoses in old age, 148
3,4-dihydroxyphenylalanine (DOPA), 139
disability (*see also* social disability)
  and alternatives to hospital care, 30
  complex of factors contributing to, 212
  Cooper's taxonomic hierarchy, 212–13, 214–15
  definition of, 210–11; changes in, 212
Disability Assessment Schedule, hierarchy of social disability using, 213
diuretics inducing psychoses in old age, 148
DOPA (3,4-dihydroxyphenylalanine), 139
dopamine, 118
drug abuse
  care facilities, 29
  long-stay patients, 185 (Fig. 1)
  in Norway, 16, 17 (Table 2)
drug therapy (*see also* antidepressants; neuroleptic drugs *and specific agents*)
  in combination with family therapy, 80
  duration of, 129–30, 134
  problems of diagnosis after, 10–11
  for psychotic children, 141
  side effects of, 55; lithium, 110; neuroleptics, 53, 68, 104–5; pharmacotoxic psychoses, 147–8

elderly (*see also* aging), 145–9
  distinction between functional and non-functional psychoses, 146
  factors affecting psychoses in, 145–6; cerebral functioning, 145–6; experience, 146; immediate environment, 145; physical health, 146; predispositions/personality traits, 146; socioeconomic, 145
  functional psychoses appearing in, 147
  incidence of chronic illness in, 177
  pharmacotoxic psychoses, 147–8
  psychoses in, 10, 145–9
electro-convulsive therapy (ECT)
  compared with antidepressants, 115
  in schizophrenia, efficacy of, 62, 63
  and suicide rates, 238–9
environment
  physical, and relapse in schizophrenia, 128–9
  and psychosis in old age, 145
European Medical Research Councils (EMRC), 3
expectations of patients, nurses and family, and success of rehabilitation, 132
expressed emotion (EE) of relatives, 241–5
  assessment of, 244–5
  in depressive neurosis, 243, 244
  and maintenance of weight loss by obese women, 243
  in manic-depressive psychosis, 243–4
  and non-relatives, influence of, 243
  and other measures of family functioning, 245

expressed emotion (EE) (*cont.*)
  and schizophrenic relapse, 72–3, 163, 241; cultural differences in, 242; social intervention trials, 72–3, 127–8, 241–2, 243
  and skin conductance changes in schizophrenia, 69–70

family
  aggression and psychotic relapse, 94
  analysis of costs of mental illness to, 249–50
  care (*see also* home care), 31, 195
  expectations, and success of rehabilitation, 132
  expressed emotion, *see* expressed emotion of relatives
  functioning, measures of, 245
  interactions, 241–5
  investigation of, 82–3
  psychogenic, 139
  role in development of schizophrenia, 79, 80
family doctors, *see* general practitioners
family therapy
  for correction of social networks, 171
  for psychotic children, 141
  for schizophrenia, 77–86, 128; in combination with drug therapy, 80; conjoint family therapy, 79, 85; couple therapy, 85; development of, 79–80; encountering and supportive conjoint therapy, 79, 83–5 (Fig. 2); Finnish multicentre project involving, 80–6; individual therapy and, 86; investigation of family situation before, 82–3; need for, 78–9; support for the family, 85–6; system-orientated therapy, 80, 85
family-care homes (*see also* home care), 31
Finland
  development of treatment of new schizophrenics, 80–6
  mental health services in, 151
  rehabilitation of schizophrenics, 152–61
Finnish Form for Schizophrenics' Families (FFSF), 82–3
Fould's Symptom–Sign Inventory (SSI), 222, 223, 224
functional psychoses (*see also* chronic psychotics *and specific psychoses*)
  case registers for monitoring treatment outcome, 197–205
  in childhood and adolescence, 139–43
  classification of, 11–13
  definition of, 9–10
  incidence of, 177–8
  long-term treatment of (*see also* long-term treatment): alternatives to hospital, 30–2; in Italy, 39–46; milieu therapy, 89–98; with neuroleptics, 101–5; optimum duration of, 51–5
  numbers of admissions, in Norway, 16, 17 (Table 2)
  in old age, 145–9
  prevalence of, 178; in Ireland, 203
  psychological treatments for, 59–74
  suicides and, 235–9
Funen county, Denmark, suicide behaviour in, 236–8 (Fig. 1, Table 1)

General Health Questionnaire (GHQ), 222–3
general practice, incidence of endogenous depression in, 12
general practitioners
  care of chronic relapsing patients and, 221–2
  role in mental health services, 191
genetic factors in chronification of schizophrenia, 133
Geneva psychiatric case register, 200
Germany, Federal Republic of, psychiatric case registers, 200
Gröningen psychiatric case register, 199
group therapy versus individual therapy in schizophrenia, 63–4
group work in therapeutic milieus
  quality of, 97
  quantity of exposure to, 96–7

haloperidol, 103
handicaps
  definition of, 210–11
  development of, 30–1
health care policy, changes in, 178–9
heart-rate changes in schizophrenia, 69
Holland, Gröningen psychiatric case register, 199
home care for schizophrenics, 78–9, 153–4
home visits, 49, 153
homelessness and psychiatric disorder, 218, 225–6
'hospital hostel' for chronic psychotics, 227
hospitalization
  of psychotic children, 140, 142
  and rehabilitation, 151–61
  syndrome, 160
hospitals, psychiatric, *see* psychiatric hospitals *and also* psychiatric departments of general hospitals
hostel ward and mental hospital, comparison of costs of, 249, 250

hostels, 220
'hospital', for chronic psychotics, 227
long-stay patients in, 202
sociotherapeutic, 154
housing and working axes in rehabilitation, 131–2 (Fig. 4)
human leukocytic antigen (HLA) and schizophrenia, 205
hypnotherapy for schizophrenia, 73

Iceland, psychiatric reporting system in, 200
imipramine compared to phenelzine, 115
impairment(s)
definition of, 210–11
social, assessment of, 230–1
types of, 30
in-patient(s) (*see also* out-patient care; patients; psychiatric beds; psychiatric hospitals *and* psychiatric institutions)
adjustment in relation to adaptation in the community, 92
discharges of, in Italy, 47
length of stay (*see also* long-term patients): and rates of readmission, 34; time limits on, 34; trends in, 187 (Table 2)
numbers of: in Ireland, 202–3; in Norway, 15–16 (Table 1); in USA, 29 (Table 1)
services, utilization of, in Europe, 258, 259 (Table 4)
infanto-juvenile psychosis, 139–41
information systems, need for improvement of, 260
institutional neurosis, 31
institutionalism, 31
institutionalization, 220
International Classification of Diseases (ICD), 9, 11–13
International Classification of Impairments, Disabilities and Handicaps (ICIDH), 210–11
interventions, social, *see* social interventions
involuntary admissions, *see* compulsory admissions
involutional depression, 147
Ireland
prevalence rates of psychiatric illness, 203–4
psychiatric case registers, 200, 202–5
isocarboxazide
dosage required, 118
efficacy of, 116–17
Italy
closure of psychiatric hospitals in, 39–46
future developments in, 47–50
length of hospital stay in, 33–4
Lomest psychiatric case register, 200; studies using, 40–5

late schizophrenia, 147
levopromazine, 103
levothyroxin for manic-depressive psychosis, 108–9
lithium, 107–11
and carbamazepine combined treatment, 109
prophylaxis, 52–3, 107–11; alternative drugs, 108–9; non-compliance, 110–11; predictors of response to, 107–8; psychotherapy supplementing, 109–10
side-effects, 110
Local Authorities, provision of community services by, 220
Lomest psychiatric case register, 200
studies utilizing, 40–5
long-term patients (*see also* chronic psychotics; new long-stay patients *and* old long-stay patients)
characteristics of, 16–17
'code' of chronicity, 100
diagnostic composition of, 185–6 (Fig. 1)
in Italy, 39–40
long-term treatment (*see also* community care; chronic psychotics *and specific treatments*)
of adolescents, 141–2
of children, 140–1
classification of functional psychoses requiring, 9–13
continuity of, 128, 129, 221
cost–effectiveness analysis, 247–54
a definition of, 51
with lithium, *see* lithium prophylaxis
milieu therapy, 89–98
with monoamine oxidase inhibitors (MAOIs), 119
with neuroleptics (*see also under* neuroleptic drugs), 101–5
optimum duration of, 51–5, 134
policies on, 179–80

Manchester Schizophrenia Study, 248–9, 250
manic-depressive psychosis
expressed emotion of relatives and, 243–4
lithium prophylaxis, 52–3, 107–11; alternative drugs, 108–9; non-compliance, 110–11; predictors of response to, 107–8; psychotherapy supplementing, 109–10
suicide risk, 236

Mannheim
evaluation of the community mental health service, 184–95
psychiatric case register, 184–5, 200
Marplan, *see* isocarboxazide
mental health centres, in Finland, 151, 152, 157 (Fig. 1)
Mental Health Programme of WHO, 255
mental health servies
cost-effectiveness analysis, 205, 247–54
European pilot studies on, 258–60 (Table 4)
in Finland, 151
in Italy, patterns of care, 48–50
need for a glossary and definition of terms, 260
planning, role of case registers, 202
policies on, 25, 27–8, 179–80, 255
quality of, indicators of, 251
trends in consumption, 255–60
in United Kingdom, 218–19, 220
mental hospitals, *see* psychiatric hospitals
Mental Illness Research, Study Group on, 3
mental retardation
care facilities, 28
life expectancy in, 178
long-stay patients, 185 (Fig. 1)
Middlesex Hospital Questionnaire, 223
milieu therapy, 89–98
design of studies on, 91–2, 95–7
development of, 90–1
differentiation of wards, 20, 21, 23
efficacy of, 62–3, 91
group exposure: quality of, 97; quantity of, 96–7
measurement of variables of, 92–3, 95
percentage of psychotic patients, 97
therapeutic characteristics of effective, 93–5
and types of psychoses, 97–8
monoamine oxidase, types A and B, 117
monoamine oxidase inhibitors (MAOIs), 115–20
brain neurotransmitters and, 118–19
chemical specificity of, 117
dosage, 118
long-term therapy, 119
metabolism of, 118
type of depression responding to, 115–17
morbidity, assessment of, 222–3
multiaxial diagnostic systems, 103
mute patient, reinstitution of speech in, 67
mutism induced by phenothiazines, 68

neglect of patients
after discharge in Italy, 47
chronic psychotics, 217–31
in psychiatric hospitals, 226
neuroleptic drugs
for affective psychoses, 52
development of new, 103–4
efficacy of, 102–3, 127
inducing psychoses in old age, 148
long-term treatment with, 101–5; need for treatment programmes, 104; optimum duration of, 53–4, 68
monitoring of, 105
for paranoid states, 54
side effects, 53, 68, 104–5
neurotic depression
classification of, 12
critical attitudes of relatives in, 243, 244
neurotic disorders
long-stay patients, 185 (Fig. 1)
in Norway, 16, 17 (Table 2)
prevalence rates in Ireland, 203
response to phenelzine in, 116
neurotic symptoms of psychotic patients, 223
neurotransmitters and MAOIs, 118–19
new long-stay patients, 152
accumulation of, 202; in Italy, 43–4; in Mannheim, 185, 188 (Fig. 3)
comparison of costs of services for, 249
diagnostic composition of, 185–6 (Fig. 1)
research needs, 253
noradrenaline CSF values in depression, 118
North Häme, Finland, mental health care services, 152
Norway, structural changes in psychiatric hospitals in, 15–23
Nottingham psychiatric case register, 198
Novi, case register studies in, 40–3
nurses, community psychiatric, costs of, compared with out-patient care, 249
nursing care, patients requiring, 21
nursing homes, psychiatric, in Norway, 17–18 (Table 3)
nursing staff (*see also* staff of psychiatric hospitals)
expectations of, and success of rehabilitation, 132
psychiatric, undesirable effects of, 67

obese women, critical attitudes of relatives and maintenance of weight loss by, 243
old long-stay patients
declining numbers of, in Italy, 43 (Fig. 2); in Mannheim, 185, 188 (Fig. 3)
diagnostic composition of, 185–6 (Fig. 1)
organic psychoses, 10
numbers of in-patients, in Norway, 16, 17 (Table 2)

out-patient care (*see also* community care *and* in-patients)
  costs of, compared with community psychiatric nurses, 249
  in Finland, 151, 153
  in Italy, 48, 49
  patterns of utilization by schizophrenics, 190–1 (Fig. 5)
  problems of treatment adherence, 69
  utilization of, in Europe, 258, 259 (Table 4)
outcome
  assessment of, for cost–effectiveness analysis, 250
  case registers for monitoring, 201–2, 203–4
  social network variables as a measure of, 168–9
Oxford psychiatric case register, 199
Oxford record linkage project, 198

paranoid psychoses, classification of, 12, 13
paranoid states, duration of long-term treatment for (*see also* delusional states), 54
paraphrenia, 12, 147
pargyline, selectivity of, 117
Parkinson's syndrome, psychoses in, 148
patients (*see also* chronic psychotics *and* in-patients)
  access to records, 73, 201
  appropriateness of care provided, 18–19
  attitudes to drug side effects, 104–5
  census of, in Norway, 17–18 (Table 3)
  compliance, *see* compliance
  continuity of care, 128, 129, 221
  Data Protection Laws and, 200–1
  expectations, and success of rehabilitation, 132
  long-term, *see* long-term patients
  neglect of, *see* neglect of patients
  perceptions of therapeutic milieus: assessment of, 92–3; of effective milieus, 93–4
  'revolving door', 44
  self-rating by, 223
  suicide by, 236, 237–8 (Fig. 1, Table 1); registration of, 236
  types of, 13
  views on structural changes in psychiatric hospitals, 22
Patients' Rights Movement, 60, 73
perphenazine, 103
personal construct theory, 67–8
personality disorders, long-stay patients, 185 (Fig. 1)
personality traits and psychoses in old age, 146
pharmacotherapy, *see* drug therapy
pharmacotoxic psychoses in old age, 147–8
phenelzine
  dosage required, 118
  efficacy of, 115, 116, 117
  for neurotic patients, 116
phenothiazines, mutism induced by, 68
pimozide, 103
platelet-MAO inhibition by MAOIs, 118
Present State Examination, 223
privacy of individuals and Data Protection Laws, 200–1
private care in Norway, 16, 18 (Table 3)
psychiatric beds (*see also* in-patients)
  long-term occupied, 188–9 (Fig. 3)
  per 1000 population: trends in, 257 (Table 3); variations in, 10
psychiatric case registers, *see* case registers
psychiatric departments of general hospitals, 33–4
  'catchment areas', 221
  cost-effectiveness analysis of, 252–3
  increase in numbers of, 256–7 (Table 2)
  in Italy (*see also* Diagnosis and Treatment Services), 33–4, 39
  length of stay, 34, 219, 229
  in Norway, 17, 18 (Table 3)
  in United Kingdom, 218, 219, 220
psychiatric homes
  numbers of residents in, 186 (Fig. 1), 187–8
  proportion of long-stay patients in, 188–9 (Fig. 3)
psychiatric hospitals (*see also* in-patients)
  alternatives to (*see also* community care), 25–36, 258
  appropriateness of placement of patients, 18–19
  closure of: in Italy, 39–46, 47; some problems caused by, 35–6
  cost comparisons with hostel wards, 249, 250
  declining populations of (*see also* deinstitutionalization), 15–16 (Table 1), 27–8, 29 (Table 1), 186–7 (Fig. 2)
  diagnostic composition of patients in, 16–17 (Table 2), 185–6 (Fig. 1)
  future of, 33, 226–7
  history of development of, 26–7, 179
  neglect in, 226
  in Norway, 15–23; evaluation of structural changes in, 19–22; survey and census of, 15–18
  patterns of utilization by schizophrenics, 186–90 (Figs. 2–4, Tables 1 and 2)
  reduction in numbers of large (more than 1000 beds), 255–6 (Table 1)
  research needs, 23

psychiatric hospitals (*cont.*)
social control function of, 27, 33, 34–5
staff, *see* staff of psychiatric hospitals
structural changes in, 15–23, 35
wards, need for differentiation of, 20, 21, 23
psychiatric institutions
census investigations *see* census investigations
new long-stay, in Italy, 48
variations in use of, 10
psychiatric nursing homes, in Norway, 17–18 (Table 3)
psychiatric services, *see* mental health services
psychiatrists, numbers of, 258
psychoanalysis, 60
psychogenic family, 139
psychological treatments (*see also* psychotherapy), 59–74
psychometric tests, 222–3
psychophysiological techniques in schizophrenia, 69–70
psychoses (*see also* chronic psychoses; functional psychoses *and specific psychoses*), 9
organic causes of, 139–40
problems of identifying, 223–4
suicide risk, 236, 238
psychosocial factors in chronic schizophrenia, 133
psychotherapy, 59–74
for affective psychoses, 53
as an alternative to long-term drug therapy, 68
classifications and definitions, 60
compliance with research protocol, 70
evaluation of, 60–1
plus lithium for manic-depressive psychoses, 109–10
as prophylaxis in children, 71–2
psychodynamic, 60
of psychogenic family, 139
for psychotic children, 141
for schizophrenia, 59, 61–2; efficacy of, 62–3; group *v* individual therapy, 63–4; the therapists' variable, 63

quality of life of chronic patients, 4
after rehabilitation, 159
assessment of, 70–1
quality service, indicators of, 251

rating scales, 223
rational-emotive therapy, 64
reactive psychoses, classification of, 13
readmissions
increasing frequency of, 186–7 (Table 1)
predictors of, 190
records, access of patients to, 73, 201
rehabilitation, 130–2
development of an integrated system in Finland, 154–61
effect of age on success of, 159
home care experiment, 153–4
housing and working axis, 131–2 (Fig. 4)
potential of hospitalized patients, 152, 159
sociotherapy in a small community, 154
relapse (*see also* expressed emotion of relatives and schizophrenic relapse)
and family aggression, 94
prevention of, social network interventions for, 170–2
social network variables and, 169–70
relatives, *see* family
Repertory Grid Test, Bannister's, 67–8
Revealed Differences Technique, 245
'revolving door' patients, in Italy, 44

St Loman's psychiatric case register, 202
Salford psychiatric case register, 199
schizoaffective psychoses, classification of, 11
schizophrenia
acute: classification of, 11; milieu therapy for, 93
aetiology of, family factors in, 79, 80
after adolescent psychosis, 141
age-related incidence rates, 177–8
aging and, 148–9
chronic: aging in, 148–9; defects, nature of, 72, 132–3; genetic factors and, 133; levels of disability, 30–1; problems of identifying, 224; psychosocial factors in, 133; social networks in, 168–9
classification of, 11
external sociofamilial structure and internalized mental concepts, 129
family therapy for, *see* family therapy for schizophrenia
homelessness and, 225–6
and human leukocytic antigen (HLA), 205
in Ireland, 203–5
late, 147
long-term care of, 31–2, 183–95
models of: illness, 78 (Fig. 1); long-term evolution, 125, 126 (Figs. 2 and 3); three-phase, 124–5 (Fig. 1)
physical environment, importance of, 128–9
prevalence, 178; rates in Ireland, 203, 204
psychophysiological techniques, 69–70
rehabilitation: development of an integrated system in Finland, 154–61;

effect of age on success of, 159; home care experiment, 153–4; potential of hospitalized patients, 152, 159; social and vocational, 127, 130–2; sociotherapy in a small community, 154
relapse: expressed emotion of relatives and, *see under* expressed emotion of relatives; modification of social networks and, 171–2; prevention of acute, 127–8; social network variables as risk factors in, 169–70
sex differences in aftercare, 192
social disability and impaired cognitive abilities, 209
suicide risk, 236
syndromes I and II, 127, 134
thought disorders of: personal construct theory and, 67–8; and social networks, 172–3
treatment, 123–35; continuity of, 128; drugs, duration of treatment, 53–4, 129–30, 134; further research needs, 129; hypnotherapy, 73; milieu therapy (*see also* milieu therapy), 91–8; psychotherapy, 59–60, 61–3; self-instructional training, 66; simplification of informational input, 128; social skills training in, 66–7
Schizophrenia Study, Manchester, 248–9, 250
self-esteem, growth of, in community groups, 160
self-help organizations, 171
self-instructional training, 64–5, 66
self-rating scales, 223
senile delusional states, 147
senile depression, 147
senile psychoses, numbers of patients, in Norway, 16, 17 (Table 2)
serotonin, 118
Sestri, case register studies in, 40–3
sex differences in aftercare received by schizophrenics, 192
sheltered homes, 190 (Table 3)
sheltered workshops, 190 (Table 3), 220
skin conductance changes in schizophrenia, 69–70
social breakdown syndrome, 4, 31
social contacts, 165
social control, psychiatric hospitals as a means of, 27, 33, 34–5
social disability (*see also* disability), 207–13
course of, 207–9 (Figs. 1 and 2)
models of, 211–13
social impairment, assessment of, 230–1
social integration as a measure of outcome, 168
social interventions, 49
in social networks, 170–2
to reduce expressed emotion of relatives, 72–3, 127–8, 241–2, 243
social network, 163–73
of chronic schizophrenics, 168–9
concept of, 164–6
definitions of, 164
intervention/prevention studies, 167 (Fig. 2), 170–2
outcome studies, 167 (Fig. 2), 168–9
problems of collecting information on, 172
risk factor studies, 167 (Fig. 2), 169–70
role of cognitive disorders in, 172–3
structural characteristics, 166 (Fig. 1)
sub-networks, 165 (Table 2)
terminology of, 164 (Table 1)
zones of intimacy, 165–6
social relationships
and cognitive disorders, 173
evaluation of quality of, 166
protective and stressful aspects of, 163–4
social skills training, 66–7, 127
socioeconomic factors in psychosis in old age, 145
sociotherapeutic hostels, 154
Sopimusvuori Association, 155–61
Southampton psychiatric case register, 199
staff of psychiatric hospitals (*see also* nursing staff)
perceptions of milieus, 92–3
satisfaction with structural changes, 21–2
Staff Resident Interaction Chronograph (SRIC), 92
applicability, 95
Study Group on Mental Illness Research, 3
suicide, 235–9
behaviour, trends in, 235, 236
high-risk groups for, 235–6
as a 'human right', 239
rates in Funen, Denmark, 237 (Fig. 1)
registration of, 236
risk and changes in therapy, 238–9
sweat-gland activity in schizophrenia, 69
Switzerland, Geneva psychiatric case register, 200
symptom-rating scales, 223
as measures of outcome of treatment, 250
Symptom–Sign Inventory, Fould's (SSI), 222, 223, 224

telephones, role in treatment of chronic psychotics, 69
therapeutic community (*see also* milieu therapy)

therapeutic community (*cont.*)
  proper, 90, 94–5
  psychiatric ward as, 23, 90
thioridazine, 103
thought disorders of schizophrenia
  personal construct theory and, 67–8
  and social networks, 172–3
Three County psychiatric case register, 202
thyroid hormone for manic-depressive psychosis, 108–9
time out from positive reinforcement (TO), 64
token economies (TE), 67
transinstitutionalization, 29
treatment, long-term, *see* long-term treatment
treatment programmes
  continuity of, 128, 129
  development of, 104

United Kingdom
  case registers, 198–9
  mental health services, 218–19, 220
'unity psychoses', 11

Ward Atmosphere Scale (WAS), 92–3
  applicability, 95
wards, need for differentiation of, 20, 21, 23
Worcester psychiatric case register, 199
working and housing axes in rehabilitation, 131–2 (Fig. 4)
World Health Organization (WHO)
  International Classification of Diseases (ICD), 9, 11–13
  International Classification of Impairments, Disabilities, and Handicaps (ICIDH), 210–11
  pilot study of European mental health services, 205, 258–60
  policy on development of mental health services, 255